SEXTASY

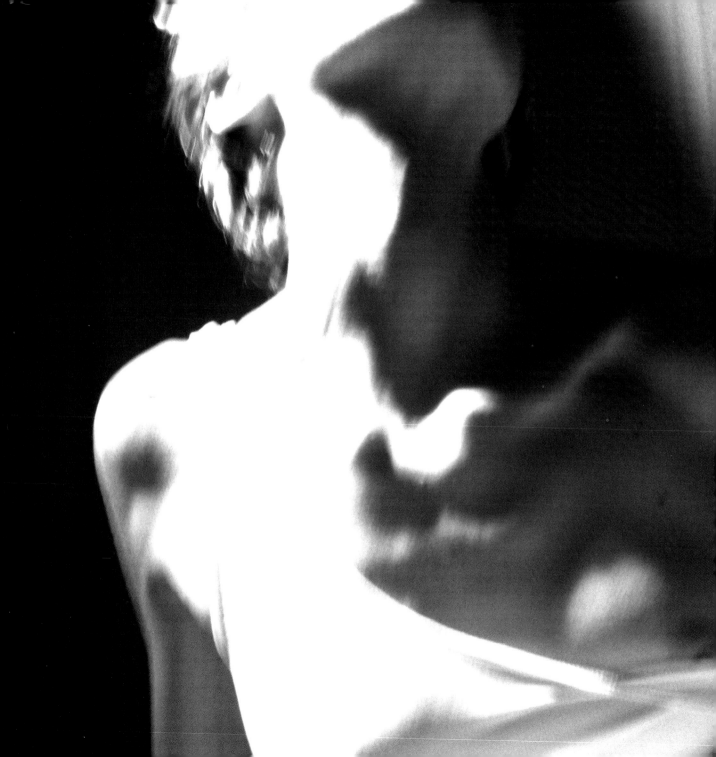

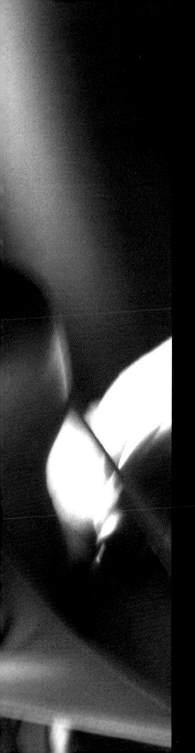

SEXTASY

MASTER THE TIMELESS TECHNIQUES OF
TANTRA, TAO, AND THE KAMA SUTRA TO TAKE
LOVEMAKING TO NEW HEIGHTS

CAROLINE ALDRED

DELTA TRADE PAPERBACKS

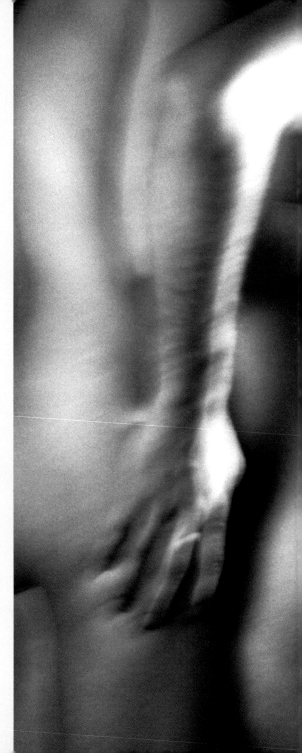

For Ashu With Love

SEXTASY
A Delta Book

PUBLISHING HISTORY
Carroll & Brown trade paperback edition published 2003
Delta trade paperback edition/February 2005

Published by
Bantam Dell
A Division of Random House, Inc.
New York, New York

Editor: Ian Wood
Designer: Frank Cawley
Photographer: Jules Selmes

Library of Congress Cataloging-in-Publication information is
available from the publisher.

ISBN 0-385-33882-1

Printed in Singapore
Published simultaneously in Canada

10 9 8 7 6 5 4 3 2 1

Cover photo © Barnaby Hall/Photonica

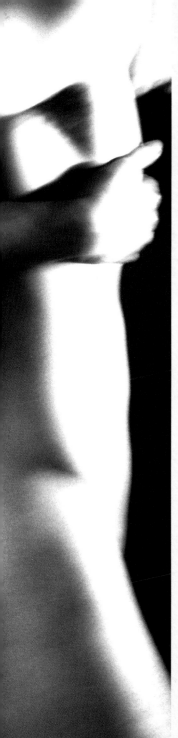

CONTENTS

INTRODUCTION

This is a book about love and sex and learning how, by bringing love into our sexual practices, we can transform and enrich ourselves and our lovers. Love is a phenomenon and sex is a mystery, and I am captivated and intrigued by them both.

Interest in sex is as old as human life, and still it holds its mysterious quality even within the limitations of our conditioned lives. Love is a phenomenon that defies definition, and we all yearn for it and seek it, and hope to share it, give it, and receive it. In fact, love is such an important and vital source of energy in our lives that it contributes enormously to our mental, emotional, spiritual, and physical well-being.

Whatever your age, gender, sexual orientation, relationship status, and religious, spiritual, or cultural persuasion, I invite you to learn how to expand your sexual and loving consciousness. By doing so, you may bring changes into your life and your values that will positively affect all aspects of your daily life, not just your sex life.

You do not need to wait for your lover to join you in order to start practice and awareness. Begin with yourself, and sooner rather than later your lover will be attracted to your discovery. Develop the relationship you have with yourself, your self-worth, self-acceptance, and your higher self, your inherent divinity. The more comfortable you are with your own sexuality, the more sexy you feel, and the more sexy you will be. The more capable you are of truly loving yourself, the more loving you will feel, and the more loving you will be.

Discover sex as dynamic meditation or experience it as a form of still meditation, alone or with a lover, in a peaceful, expressive, focused, electric, and enlightening way. Love is the spirit of sex and sex is the body of love. Sex is a journey with no destination. Love and loving is a way of being, a practice of remaining open, a practice of service as the highest honor.

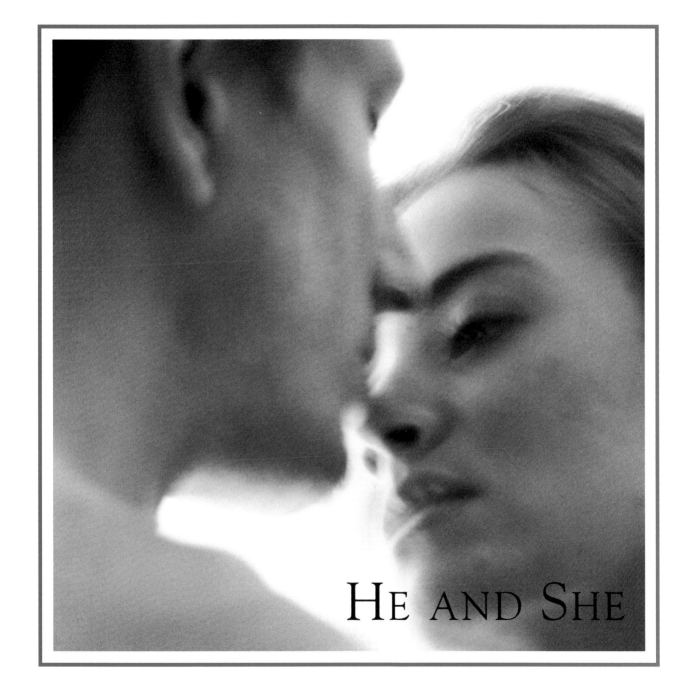

HE AND SHE

COMMITMENT

"Marriage under the Law of Shiva is of two kinds. One is terminated at the conclusion of the rite, and the other is lifelong. Both require a high level of commitment. When it is stated aloud, 'Approve our marriage according to the Law of Shiva,' a marriage commitment is truly made."

MAHANIRVANA TANTRA

Human beings all seek love from one source or another. In fact, we need love in order to survive. We have a need to receive it and a need to give it. Love is caring, both caring about and caring for. It is also communicating, and wanting to be together and to do things together, not just the daily tasks but playing, relaxing, and lovemaking as well. It requires a certain kind of openness and trust, a willingness to be vulnerable, and in that vulnerability lies great strength.

Emotions are more enduring than feelings; they can last a lifetime. That is why the arousal of the emotion of love in an intimate relationship involves a commitment and allows an opportunity for deep, shared intimacy to develop.

Whether formal or informal, any commitment motivated by true love strengthens a relationship and gives it meaning. Commitment implies absolute trust, profound acceptance, and mutual service, agreeing to give the most of ourselves to one another.

Commitment between lovers develops gradually. It is much more than sharing responsibilities such as mortgage payments, maintaining and running a home, and taking care of children. In a relationship of love, the emotional commitment to one another, and to one another's needs and emotional well-being, has to be regularly expressed and reaffirmed and thereby renewed.

Once established, commitment creates a bond that keeps the lovers together, and that bond can help them to overcome any difficulties by providing an element of strength for them to draw upon. The commitment is not simply to endure as a couple, but to make the relationship much more complete by continually exploring and renewing it.

COMMUNICATION
Communication, and learning how to communicate, is vital in any loving relationship. We all need to be cared for, comforted, loved, caressed, adored, and worshiped, but in order to receive these "blessings" we have to be willing to give them. So unless you know what your

lover likes, wants, or needs, and what he or she expects or hopes for from you, you cannot give it.

You have to be willing to listen and become aware of your lover's needs, without judging them and without feeling criticized or inadequate. Be open to your lover's desires rather than being consumed by your own. To give open-heartedly and unconditionally without expecting something in return is hard, but by giving in that way you will be rewarded. Giving can be the most rewarding of all experiences. Honoring your lover by giving the time and energy he or she requires is a very special gift.

HOW TO ASK FOR IT

It's important that you each express your wants and needs in a positive, compassionate, and empathetic way, especially when discussing your sexual desires. Suggest new ways of doing things rather than saying "I don't like it when you..." Focus on what you do like and want to experiment with. In this way you can also gauge your lover's reactions to your suggestions.

If you have difficulty expressing yourself verbally about certain things, such as what you want your lover to do for you, or what you want to do but have never dared ask for, write them down. Do this together, and always be honest and open with one another.

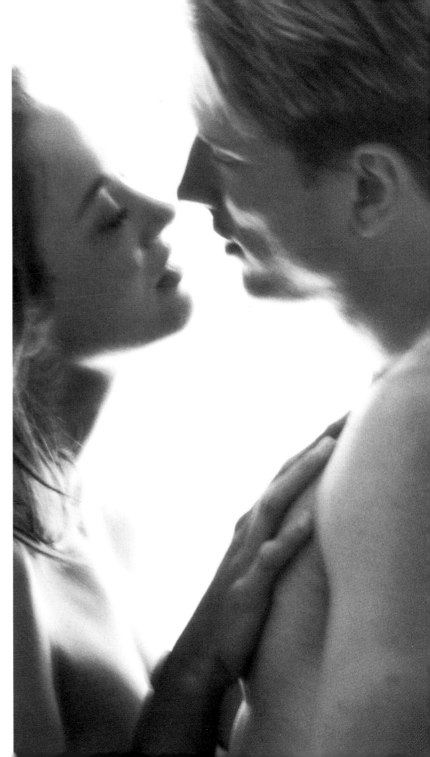

FINDING A LOVER FOR YOU

When you are hoping to find a lover you first have to believe in your own "lovability," and that comes from loving yourself and accepting yourself fully for who you really are. Love yourself, love giving love, love receiving it, and you will have a better chance of attracting your perfect lover. If you have an air of need or desperation about you, you may attract a lover, but he or she may not be one who wants a long-term, loving relationship of equals.

To be available for love also means letting go of any hurt and pain caused by a previous relationship. Wounds from an old relationship can create blockages that make it difficult to allow new love in. You need to allow yourself to feel all those painful feelings of rage, anger, fear, and grief to get them out of your body and mind. Let go and open yourself and your heart to new beginnings.

Be grateful for having had your heart broken, because it has broken your heart open and allowed you to feel. Being in touch with and sensitive to your feelings is an important aspect of loving—both loving yourself and being able to love someone else.

Only when you can love and value the person you are today will you attract other people. And those people will include that special someone who can help you to develop and grow in the direction you need.

BODY LANGUAGE

Words are not always the most effective or loving way to signal desire. Nonverbal signals, not always consciously given, can be clearer indicators of someone's interest in you or your interest in them. There are many different body language signals, some more subtle than others, that can indicate whether or not a person is interested in or attracted to you. Facial expressions, body movements, and tone of voice can all be clues to sexual interest.

Body language is the real indication of what is happening inside you, and between yourself and other people. No matter what you say, the real message is reflected in what your body does.

For example, when you are depressed or "carrying the weight of the world on your shoulders," your shoulders automatically sag and your back becomes rigid instead of being flexible. When you are tense and bottling up your emotions, your tummy muscles tighten and your walk becomes jerky. Tension affects the way you stand and the way you hold your body and the way you move. People who are open and unembarrassed will talk to you with movements of their arms, facing you. Shy people or strangers tend to avert their faces, and may also cross their arms in front of their bodies as a form of defence or protection.

THE EYES

You can learn a lot about what another person thinks of you by looking into their eyes. If someone dislikes you, the pupils of their eyes tend to narrow when they look at you. But when someone is attracted to you, his or her pupils will widen and grow. At the same time, their blink rate might increase. Most people usually blink about twice a second, but when they are sexually attracted to someone their blink rate goes up. So to find out if someone is interested in you, look into his or her eyes. If the pupils grow, there is interest. And if the blink rate goes up, be bold!

Another useful clue lies in the way the other person looks at you. As two people get to know one another, they take each other's faces in as they chat. The eyes meet, just long enough to register, and then move to the mouth, cheeks, and hair. A man interested in a woman will also tend to trace her figure with his eyes, and women do the same with men.

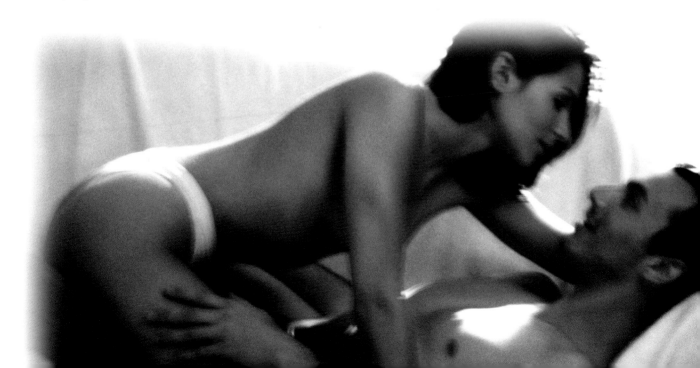

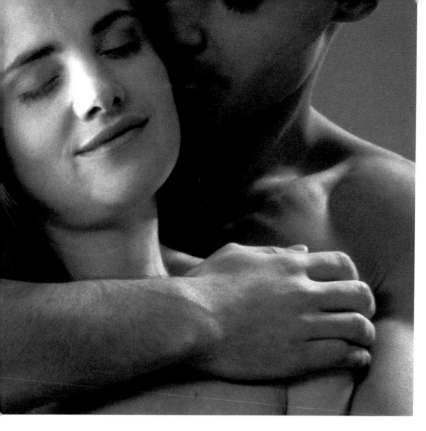

really joyful. Picture it and feel the smile coming. Now open your eyes and let your lips part, your eyes crinkle, and the edges of your mouth curl up. You might be laughing by now!

A real smile involves the muscles from around your mouth and lips to those right up to your eyes. So powerful is the smile from the heart that if you smile genuinely at someone, you will get an immediate and positive response.

When someone laughs with you or at your remarks or jokes, it is a particularly appealing signal that they are enjoying your company and it is reasonably easy to tell a false laugh from a genuine one. Over-enthusiastic laughter can, however, be a real turn-off!

TOUCHING

When someone you are talking with makes gentle physical contact, such as by touching your arm, it could be just a friendly gesture or it could mean they are attracted to you. More intimate actions, such as picking a hair or fluff from your clothing, or leaning a knee against yours under the table, are usually more reliable signs that the other person is attracted to you.

THE POWER OF ATTRACTION

People tend to be attracted to those whose physical attractiveness is comparable to their own. We expect to

SMILING AND LAUGHING

Smiling not only makes you feel better and happy, it makes you look better too. Happy, joyful, smiley people are always more attractive than sad, unhappy, depressed people. Your happiness shows in your appearance, the way you hold yourself and the energy you project.

To see how you look when you are smiling with genuine happiness, rather than forcing a smile, try this simple exercise. Look into a mirror, close your eyes, and remember the happiest time of your life or a time when you felt feel more comfortable, and less apprehensive of rejection, by choosing someone on the same level of attractiveness as ourselves.

When two people meet, the obvious initial attraction is visual. Recent research also indicates that we are attracted to one another by smell, by the scent of one another. We then use tactics such as conversation and increasingly close physical contact to reinforce the mutual attraction.

When you walk into a room and meet someone that you are attracted to, someone who excites and arouses you, you will notice that within minutes your energy perks up. Your heart beats faster, your palms may sweat, and you feel sexually aroused.

These effects are caused by the hormone epinephrine (adrenaline), produced by the body to prepare it for physical action. The rush of epinephrine makes us feel "turned on." It can lead us to mistake these sensations of physical excitement for love, and to start a relationship based purely on intense sexual attraction. However, there are many long-lasting loving relationships that started off based on powerful physical attraction. These lovers definitely fell in lust before creating an enduring bond.

Other body chemicals associated with sexual attraction include endorphins—the "pleasure chemicals"—and pheromones, substances emitted by the body to stimulate or attract a member of the opposite sex.

The production of these chemicals increases when a person is sexually aroused or in love, and they trigger very distinct biochemical changes. When lovers talk about the chemistry between them, they are right!

SOME QUESTIONS THAT MAY HELP YOU

- Am I attracted to this person because I am seeking a partner as a lover, helpmate, friend, and companion on my spiritual journey? Or am I attracted to this person because I need someone to rescue me, make me feel important, and provide security or a sexual high?

Very often, the latter goes together with the fairy-tale fantasies and illusory dreams of being "in love" forever, and together for ever and ever.

- Am I operating from hormones or heart, instinct or wisdom, or a combination of all of these?

When we create a mindful, loving connection with someone, our bodies produce the hormone oxytocin, which contributes to the feelings of sensual closeness and trust. It takes nearly four years of a reciprocal, loving union for our bodies to learn to secrete oxytocin instead of creating an epinephrine high when we are with our lovers.

GOD IN EVERY MAN

The average man tends to measure how successful he is as a lover by how many women he has seduced, how many times he was able to "do it," how long he was able to maintain his erection, how soon he was able to do it again, and so on.

Making love, however, is about quality not quantity. It is about the quality of your energy, the quality of your attention and interest. What turns women on most is when they feel you are really with them, totally present and fully devoted to them so they feel cherished and adored.

Love takes practice—practice to improve your capacity to love more freely and to experience the depth of your love more fully, without limits, and even through difficult moments. Without your capacity to love, when making love you will just be like a robot and you will never feel fulfilled. Technique without warmth or emotion takes the heart out of making love.

Love your lover, melt into her warmth. Forget sexuality, forget all that goes on in your head, in your fantasies. Don't try to prove anything, because when you start trying to prove something your mind kicks in. While you are making love, forget you are a man and she is a woman.

Be open to the full spectrum of your senses and sensations. How much pleasure do you allow yourself? When you bathe or shower do you let yourself really enjoy it—or is it just a way to be clean, a means to an end? All of this can carry over into sex. If you take the means-to-an-end approach, soon there won't be an end that really satisfies.

You need to recognize the qualities of the god in yourself and embody them, and also relate to the inner man of your lover, male or female. The god in every man is also in every woman, just as the goddess in every woman is also in every man.

SKILLFUL LOVING

The ancient Taoists, while emphasizing a tender and highly sensitive attitude toward love and sex, still equally stressed the importance of skill. They understood that if you want to do something well, you must develop the proper skills. Men and women must learn to make love if they are going to be effective lovers. An unskilled lover can make a woman feel like he is simply masturbating in her yoni.

If lovemaking is near the top of your list of favorite activities, spend some time learning how to become a better lover, just as you would spend the necessary time if you wanted to improve your sporting or job skills. A little homework and regular training to tune in to and develop the muscles you use during sexual intercourse are essential. Be prepared to work out regularly, daily if possible.

Make an effort to maximize your lovemaking skills, which will improve your self-confidence as well as your own and your lover's capacity for pleasure. But remember that skill and technique do not necessarily make you a better lover. You may be a great performer, but the pleasure you give and receive may only be surface pleasure and the real depths of pleasure may escape you.

Many men who consider themselves expert lovers leave their lovers cold, because they are so preoccupied with sexual performance. If you are preoccupied with sexual performance, you cannot truly be making love.

More important than skill is what and how much you are able to feel and how present you are able to be with your lover—to experience each moment fully without a goal to achieve. To have the capacity to feel, and to express those feelings with a degree of sensitivity, is what being human is all about. Feeling deeply and sharing those feelings deeply are wonderful qualities to bring to a loving relationship.

The Tao suggests that a man develop his loving skills so that he can both satisfy and appreciate his lover and in so doing also reap the benefits. Technique is not just about thrusting and controlling ejaculation, it is also the development of all your senses so that you can appreciate and absorb the harmony of yin and yang. Lovemaking then ceases to be a mechanical urge and becomes a total experience. When you open all your senses and let your imagination be active, then you become an artist of ecstatic loving.

Taking the Lead

Some men still consider it their duty to initiate sexual activity and to have gained enough sexual expertise to pass their experience onto their lovers. Having to project a masculine image at all times keeps them from the possibility of learning. If they are expected to know all the answers, they cannot ask any questions.

Society tends to place men in the role of sexual teachers, and most women learn about sexuality from their first male lovers. So a man is burdened with the role of orchestrating the sexual act without any input from women, who are considered to be too pure, and therefore too inexperienced, to have any sexual ideals of their own. It's no wonder then that things can go wrong.

GODDESS IN EVERY WOMAN

*"Women are peonies, spring flowers, lotuses and bowers.
Women are pomegranates, peaches, melons and pearls.
Women are receptacles, crucibles, vessels and worlds.
Women are the fruit of life, the nourishing force of Nature."*

YUAN-SHIH YEH-TING CHI

In the ancient traditions of Egypt, Greece, Arabia, India, Tibet, and China, woman was considered the initiator of love, the embodiment of sensuality, and guardian of the creative potential. It is vital to restore to our natures our divine feminine spirituality, which we have lost. The divine does not mean anything unless you feel it in your body. When you don't feel it in your body, you substitute it with other things like sex, food, shopping, and other pleasures. Learn to feel the fullness of divine love deep within yourself.

The Taoists held that women are naturally energized by beauty. By nurturing this aspect of ourselves in our everyday lives, we increase our sensuality and expand our desire and sense of joy.

It is very easy, especially for women, to be consumed with the duties of home, family, and work, and to put the needs of others before our own. Our own pleasure, sexuality, desire, and personal well-being tend not to be priorities. However, we need to remember that our sexual energy is unique to us, is the very foundation of our being, and is an essential part of being fully alive.

EXERCISING YOUR SEXUALITY

Just as other aspects of our lives affect our sexuality, so our sexuality can affect every other part of our lives. A sexually satisfied woman is much happier and more optimistic, and a better lover, mother, and worker. But like anything truly worthwhile, our sexuality and sensuality require that we prioritize and make time for them. In order to have healthy and fulfilling sex lives, we need to exercise our sensuality and passion regularly, just as we exercise our bodies to keep fit and stay in shape.

A woman needs to recognize the qualities of the goddess in herself and embody them, and also relate to the inner woman of her lover, whether male or female. The god in every man is in every woman, just as the goddess in every woman is in every man.

Awaken the goddess within you and be alive to the erotic possibilities of the world around you. It is visible all around you in Nature, in art, in the

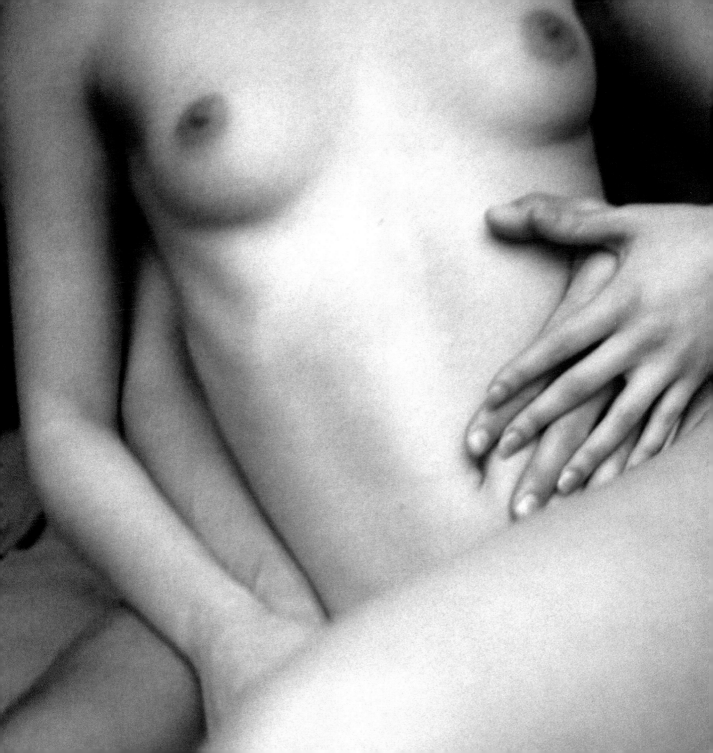

everyday things that go unnoticed but are all for your pleasure. Kindle your desire for life and sensuality, celebrate art and beauty.

Meet your inner goddess and the different aspects of her at different times. Talk to her, encourage a dialogue with her. Ask her how she would like you to dress this morning or wear your hair. Dance with her, walk with her. Ask her in what ways you should choose to pleasure yourself. It might be wearing sensual clothes that caress your skin, buying yourself flowers, listening and dancing to soft music, taking a hot and luxurious bath with special oils by candlelight, or treating yourself to the pleasure of tantalizing foods.

Honor yourself and the energy of the goddess in all things. Light a candle, make a wish, say a prayer, give thanks, offer gratitude, show appreciation. Respect yourself and who you are and your connectedness to all things—within and without, above and below.

HONORING YOUR BODY

Consider your body as a temple, a place of worship dedicated to the service of your higher self, your soul, the god and goddess within you. In the body are all the elements—space, air, fire, water, and earth. Look on your body as a temple that needs to be kept clean, healthy, and harmonious out of respect for the

divinity within. It is important to really regard the body as a temple and to worship the temple of the body as a total act of love.

It is also important to respect your personal well-being and to give priority to your own pleasure. Begin by dedicating time each week to nurturing your sexual self, and then dedicate time to it each day. Cultivating your sexual energy will transform and increase your overall energy and vitality.

Ultimately, everyone benefits from a sexually satisfied woman—especially the woman! You will experience more optimism, more happiness, and this in turn will affect the people in your life in a more positive way. And there is no doubt that enhanced feelings of self-worth lead to more enjoyable sex and a greater capacity for love. If you feel good about yourself it manifests itself outwardly in your sexuality.

Another way to boost your sexuality is through recognizing and loving your true self. By creating some kind of ritual to suit your individual needs, you allow the time and space to reconnect with your true self and to honor the goddess within you. The following ritual, or puja, can take many forms and is a simple expression of your love and devotion. It brings you closer to the divine within, to the living goddess that is YOU.

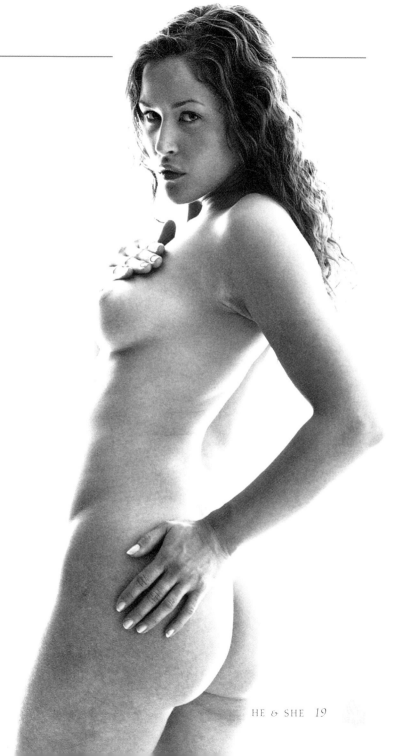

PERFORMING A PUJA

In India, people perform rituals every day for their different gods and goddesses. In the puja, they bow to their idols, offer flowers, and feed the idols with their love, because these statues represent the different aspects of the Hindu gods and goddesses.

Performing a puja to honor yourself involves offering devotional love to your own body. Stand naked in front of a mirror and say "I love you" for 15 minutes, then repeat the exercise saying first "You love me" and then "You are so beautiful."

When you bathe or take a shower, treat your body with love, honor, respect, and gratitude. When you eat, close your eyes and consider the food as an offering to your own body, to the temple where a goddess resides.

Do this ritual every day and you will feel your love for your body growing stronger and deeper each day, and you will no longer reject yourself. When you have created the perfect relationship between yourself and your body, you will no longer depend upon the success of a relationship from the outside.

Then you will be able to treat your lover's body with the same love, honor, respect, and gratitude, thus honoring the god and goddess that reside within you both.

SURRENDER

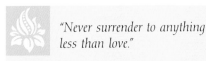

"Never surrender to anything less than love."

DAVID DEIDA

To most people, surrender is admitting defeat or yielding to the possession and power of another. There is no resistance, however, in surrendering to love. Surrender is the way to open fully and authentically to your lover and experience the most intense and profound experience of sexual loving possible. Surrender is not a sign of weakness and not all surrender is negative. If we are willing to surrender our hearts to love, then ecstasy awaits us.

When we talk about surrender in terms of loving, it is important to understand that it is about yielding to the state of love and freeing ourselves of the resistance to total openness. We have to let down our guard, be uninhibited in our feelings, be as open as we can, pull down boundaries, do away with defenses, and relinquish and abandon thought and the aspiration to prove or achieve. To experience a deep sensuality, we have to transcend emotional and physical boundaries to love beyond limits. We must yield to the moment and to the experience of love without duality. In the giving up of yourself, you can merge with another to become One.

Surrendering is not easy but it is something we can learn and practice. It feels very risky to give up our egos, our boundaries, and to trust so much that we are willing to become absolutely vulnerable. Yet vulnerability is essential if we are to give and receive with an open heart. When we no longer protect ourselves, we are open to love in its most powerful, sublime form.

LEARNING HOW TO SURRENDER

Surrendering to the moment is being fully present for a lover, letting go of all conscious thoughts and entering completely into feelings.

While making love to one another, forget all about the fact that you are man and woman, or man and man, or woman and woman. Allow the boundaries to merge and mix. For the moment, forget sexuality, forget all that goes on in your head, and just allow yourself to surrender to the life force. Float in it and melt into one another. In loving your woman, melt into her warmth; in loving your man, melt into his being.

Let go of the mind, let your body relax, and you will experience a profound sensitivity—an open heart, deep trust, and love. You need not concern yourselves with the positions of your bodies; the positions of your minds is more relevant. Just change your minds, and if you are both deeply surrendered, your bodies will take the right position that is needed in the moment. While making love there is no need to prove anything. When you do start trying to prove something, your minds take over and you are no longer in feeling mode.

For a woman to open to trust and thus surrender, she needs to feel that her lover is fully present, to feel that he is "there" without distraction, that he is relaxed and open. Only then, when she feels safe, will she open her heart and allow herself to let go completely.

For a man to allow himself to open to surrender, he needs to be directed out of his thinking mind and into his feeling body. His partner can help by using her body and presence to demonstrate uninhibited openness and heart-connected pleasure.

She should respond to her lover's loving with sighs and moans of pleasure. As she softens her body and her breath, and opens her heart and emotions, her man will respond by opening to experience a deep intimacy. The deeper the woman's surrender and her trust for her lover, the more his response will be to open with her in complete devotion.

It can take time to learn to trust and to open more to a lover's love. But there are a number of exercises you can try that will help you become closer and more intimate with each other.

USING TONGLEN

Andrew Harvey and Mark Matousek, in *Dialogues with a Modern Mystic*, suggest using Tonglen—a Tibetan meditation exercise—to make lovers more intimate. To perform Tonglen, you first breathe in and imagine that you are breathing all the pain, fear, doubt, and ignorance of your lover into your heart in the form of dark, black smoke. You pray that it will destroy all parts of your self-importance. Then when you breathe out, you imagine yourself as a wish-fulfilling jewel shedding cool light upon your beloved and giving him or her everything that is needed, psychically and emotionally.

This exercise gives each lover the opportunity to gaze deep into the other's soul—with all its sadness, imperfection, and hunger for healing— taking on all that pain and being grateful for the chance of working for the other's liberation.

To know and understand the basic truth about love, we need to recognize and accept the sacredness of sex, and accept the divinity of sex within each of us, with an open heart and an open mind. The more fully we accept sex with an open heart and mind, the freer we will be of our obsession with it. The total acceptance of life, and everything that is natural in life, will lead us to unknown heights and to pleasures that are truly sublime.

Love is a sacred art and like any art takes practice. With practice, ecstatic lovemaking becomes the rule rather than the exception.

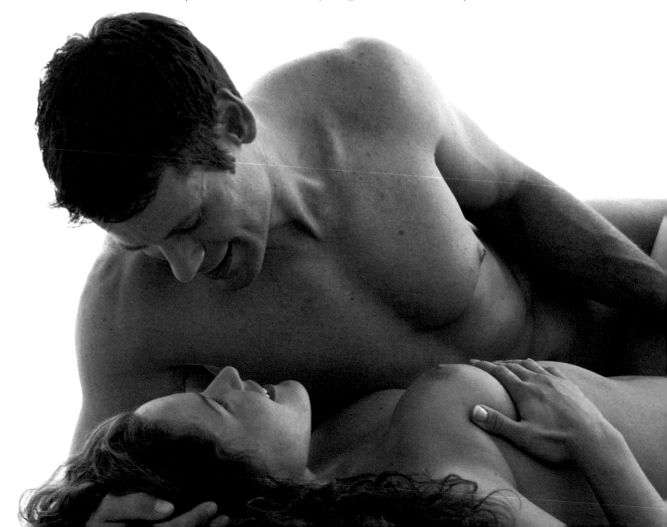

Morning/Evening "Prayers"

The following exercise has been my most moving, inspiring, erotic, and sometimes challenging experience!

The Morning and Evening "Prayers" are actually a form of meditation, combining communion with spirit, soul, and body with internal exercise and healing. The objective of performing these prayers is to achieve oneness or complete peace and harmony between oneself and one's lover. Man and woman become one perfect person. When you perform a prayer to start the day, it enlivens the body, and when you perform one to conclude the day, it relaxes the body.

The man lies on top of the woman

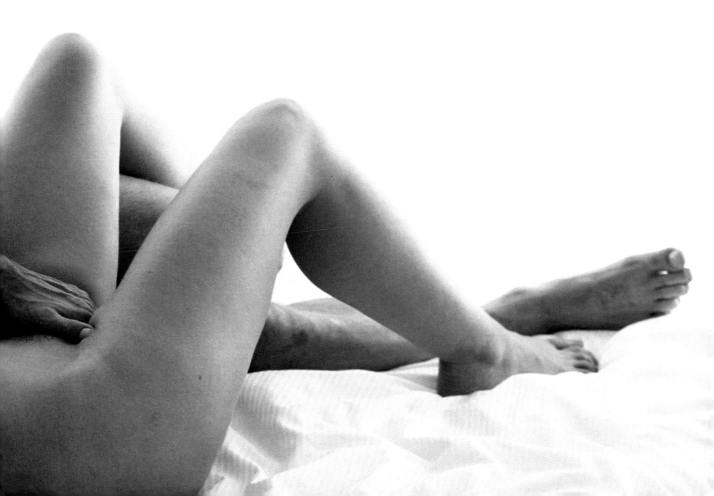

as in the missionary position. Then, with eyes closed, both partners interlock mouths, legs, and arms. The man penetrates the woman, and uses just enough movement to maintain an erection (he must be careful not to ejaculate). The couple should remain in this position for as long as they desire, so that they can enjoy and share the feelings derived from such closeness and stillness.

STANDING POSITION

This simple variation on the standing lovemaking position will help keep you

"Surrender all those ideas about being what you are not, and become what you really are. When you surrender to your nature, to what you really are, you no longer suffer. When you surrender to the real you, you surrender to life, you surrender to God. Once you surrender, there is no longer a struggle, there is no resistance, there is no suffering."

DON MIGUEL RUIZ

present in the here and now. You stand face to face, and the woman locks one leg around her lover's legs to help maintain balance.

Each of you should then place your right hand on top of your lover's head and your left hand against the small of

your lover's back. Kiss sensuously then maintain eye contact. Feel the energy being drawn upward from your feet, flowing up your legs, up your spine and into your head, and then out of the top of your head.

LISTENING TO THE HEART

Give each other the time and space to practice this exercise when one or both of you feels the need to express your feelings without criticism and without blame. It allows you to refocus yourselves away from your hurt or pain, and helps you to understand and listen to how your lover is feeling.

You sit facing each other, holding hands. Your partner takes a few minutes to explain what is upsetting him or her, while you just listen compassionately and let your heart soften. Then you repeat what you have heard. If your lover thinks there are things that you missed, invite him or her to repeat them to you.

When you've finished repeating what your lover has said to you, it is your turn to express your feelings by describing what is upsetting you. Talk about how you feel rather than what your lover has or has not done. The more vulnerable you can be with each other, the more your hearts will open and the more compassionate and positive the exercise will be.

Open your hearts and practice the exercise with a spirit of love and humility. Only with the openness of your body and your heart can you truly feel the flow of energy within you and between you and your lover.

Learn to make love from your heart. Without your sincere love for one another, sex is simply friction. Although friction sometimes feels good, only a true, genuine love will bind your bodies together in ecstatic lovemaking for a lifetime.

CONNECTING WITH LOVE

Being in love is the most exhilarating state of mind possible. When you are in love, it feels natural to gaze deeply into each other's eyes. You want to hold hands as if never to let go, to hold each other close for hours, to sit together in silence, with the feeling of closeness content just to "be" with one another.

For every couple, the high of the initial magnetism comes to an end eventually and it is easy to lose "touch" with one another. As your relationship goes through changes and evolution, do not neglect being attentive.

By gazing, holding, touching, and adoring your lover you can recapture those early feelings of being in love. And by focusing your emotional energy on each other you are creating a powerful and lasting bond between you.

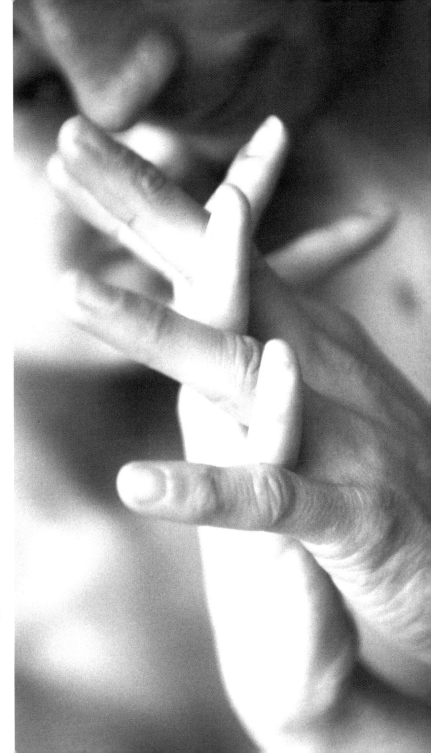

The following exercises will help you to stay connected, and you can either practice them on their own or as a part of your lovemaking. You can be naked or clothed, but you must be open and willing to share without expectations.

HEART TO HEART

This exercise will help you to feel and breathe eternity held in a moment of bliss. You sit facing each other, then you each extend your right arm and place your right palm over your lover's heart area—in the middle of his chest or in the valley between her breasts. Then you each place your left palm over the back of the other's right hand while it rests gently on your chest.

Breathe together and gaze deeply into one another's eyes. Feel your lover from your heart. Do this for several minutes and then lean toward one another and touch your foreheads together. Continue breathing together, close your eyes, and feel the energy created between you.

FINGERTIP LOVING

Remove your glasses or contact lenses, if you wear them. Sit facing each other, holding your hands up toward each other and letting just your fingertips touch. Take a few deep breaths to relax, and feel your eyes softening. After a few moments, gaze into each other's eyes,

then focus your attention on your lover's left eye. As well as gazing into your lover's eye, focus on the delicate sensations at your fingertips. Increase your awareness of the subtle energies of the body that surround and flow between you.

As you gaze into your lover's eye, repeat silently or out loud "I recognize and accept your essence." If you can manage it, practice this exercise for about twenty to thirty minutes, and then make love.

SMILE!

This is a wonderful way to practice making meaningful, heartfelt contact with your lover. Make the decision together to create a space of love energy between you as often as you can. Warmly hold your lover's hands, look steadily into one another's eyes, and smile! Stay together like this for a few minutes, gazing, holding, and smiling, and reconnect with one another in a warm and positive way.

Do not attempt to recapture the past, to repeat, copy, or imitate what has gone before. Be open to the brand-new, to all the newness and freshness and wonder and awe that life and your experiences have to offer.

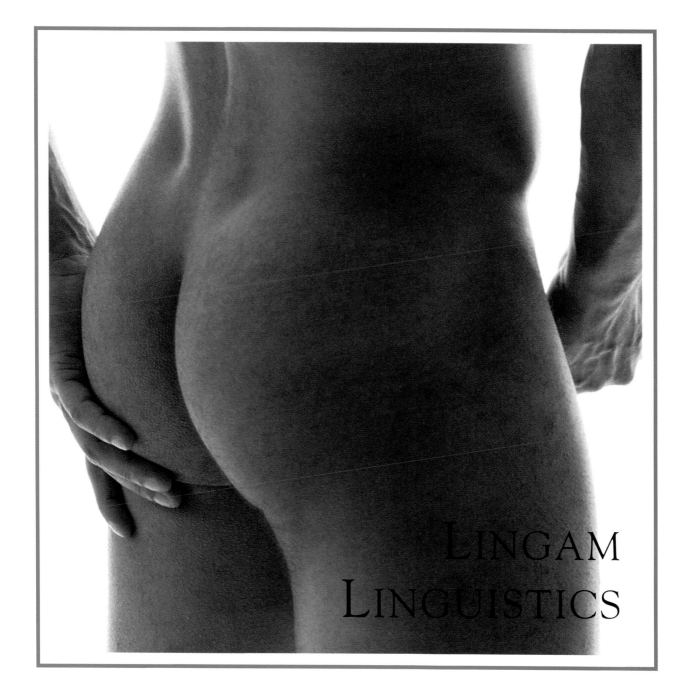

LINGAM
LINGUISTICS

THE LINGAM

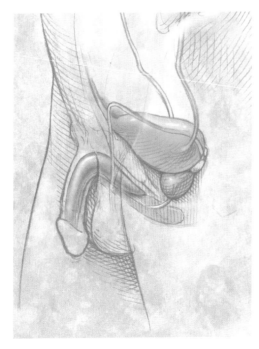

For thousands of years, many different cultures around the world have revered the lingam as a symbol of virility, courage, and power.

The word "lingam" is a Sanskrit term of reverence for the statues and images of the god Shiva's sexual organ. It is also used as a name for the penis, and I prefer to use it because it is less "biological" and also connotes the presence of the divine in the human.

The lingam has been a sacred symbol since early prehistory—the image of the creative principle, the source of life, the manifestation of virility, courage, and power. And, as such, the lingam has long been revered and worshiped by many different cultures and religions throughout the world.

The principal parts of a man's genitalia are his lingam, his testicles (testes), and his prostate gland. The lingam is made up of spongelike tissues surrounding the urethra, a thin tube that runs through its center and along which urine and semen are discharged. The two testicles are enclosed within a bag of skin called the scrotum. Each is suspended within the scrotum by a spermatic cord, a cord of tissue that supplies it with blood and nerve connections. The cord also provides a duct (the vas deferens) along which sperm passes after it has been produced by the testicle.

The vas deferens delivers the sperm to the seminal vesicles, where it mixes with the seminal fluid (semen) produced by the seminal vesicles, the prostate (see page 32), and other glands.

When a man becomes sexually aroused, the spongelike tissues of his lingam become engorged with blood, making it swell, stiffen, and become erect. As he nears ejaculation (see page 36), his testicles are drawn up toward his body, the wall of his scrotum thickens and tightens, and his blood pressure, heart rate, breathing rate, and skin temperature increase.

Rhythmic contractions of the prostate, seminal vesicles, and vas deferens pump semen into the base of the urethra. When ejaculation occurs, the semen is forced along the urethra and out of the tip of the lingam by another series of contractions, this time of the urethra and the muscles of the base and shaft of the lingam.

Although the male body may stop growing at the age of thirty, the lingam continues to grow, and it grows until a man dies. The older the man is, the bigger his lingam becomes.

Lingam Sizes and Shapes

Do not believe anyone who tells you size does not matter—it does! And it matters mostly to men. Almost all men want to have bigger lingams, no matter how large they are already. Men are often embarrassed or ashamed when they compare the size of their unerect lingams with those of other men. However, an unerect lingam is not an accurate gauge of the size of an erect one. Generally, men with larger unerect lingams experience less change in size during the transition from unerect to erect states. But men with smaller unerect lingams experience drastic changes in size during the transition from unerect to erect. The real problem with size is the importance men attach to it. And it is important, for two reasons: one is the psychological effect on the man who thinks his lingam is too small, and judges his overall worth by his size; the other is its compatibility with the size of his lover's yoni.

The perfect lingam or yoni is that which matches its counterpart perfectly. However, there are lovemaking postures that make up for any imbalance. Wide-open positions allow extra room for a large lingam to enter a small yoni comfortably, while using pillows to raise a woman's buttocks gives the man with a smaller lingam much deeper entry. Loveplay (foreplay) helps to create the high sexual arousal that is essential for counteracting major size differences, and using your hands, lips, and tongue is a lovely way to arouse your partner.

According to the Taoists, all this unnecessary worry and concern regarding size is most unfortunate because size matters very little in terms of satisfying a woman. Taoists believe that the shape is much more important. There are two main shapes—the mushroom shape, which has a large head and narrow shaft, and the triangular or pencil shape, with a small, pointed head and a wide shaft.

A mushroom-shaped lingam, when erect, is considered to be the most effective for satisfying a woman. The large head is thought to be desirable because it provides the greatest amount of stimulation. It massages the sides of the yoni and the G-spot (see page 52) thoroughly and efficiently, enhancing the pleasure she experiences and enabling her to reach her full orgasmic potential more easily.

The average vaginal channel measures four inches from the entrance of the yoni to the entrance of the uterus. It expands and contracts easily in width, but it can't change much in length and its maximum lengthways expansion is only about an inch. So a

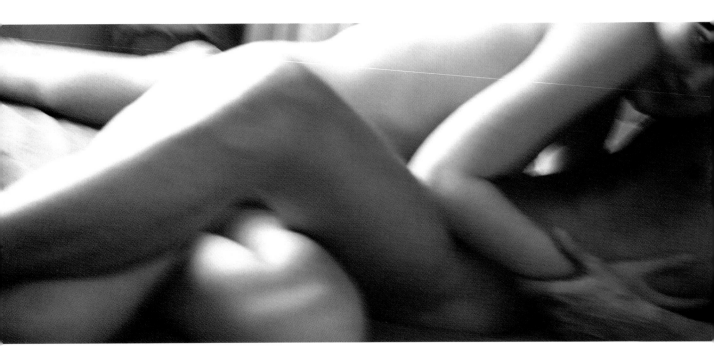

lingam that is six inches long when fully erect is the perfect match for the average-sized yoni.

If lovers are in harmony then their sex organs will adjust to fit each other. And if lovers care for each other, then it is totally irrelevant whether his lingam is long, short, thick, or thin.

Our genitals are as unique as every other part of our bodies. Accepting what nature has given us, and working with it, is infinitely more important and relevant than size and/or shape.

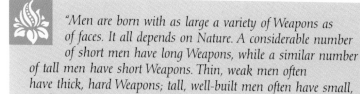

"Men are born with as large a variety of Weapons as of faces. It all depends on Nature. A considerable number of short men have long Weapons, while a similar number of tall men have short Weapons. Thin, weak men often have thick, hard Weapons; tall, well-built men often have small, weak ones."

SU-NU-MIAO-LUN

THE KAMA SUTRA'S THREE CATEGORIES OF LINGAM

THE HARE

This is the lingam that does not exceed six finger-breadths (about 5 inches) when fully erect. Usually a man with a lingam of this type is short of stature but well proportioned and of a quiet disposition. His semen is usually sweetish. He is known as being of small dimension.

THE BULL

This is the lingam that does not exceed nine finger-breadths (about 7 inches) when fully erect. A man with such a lingam is usually robust, with a high forehead, large eyes, and a restless temperament. He is ever-ready to make love and is known as being of middle dimension.

THE HORSE

This is the Lingam that is about twelve finger-breadths (about ten inches) in length when erect. The owner of such an implement is usually tall, large-framed, muscular, and has a deep voice. His nature is gluttonous, covetous, passionate, reckless, and lazy. He walks slowly and cares little for lovemaking, unless suddenly overcome by desire. His semen is copious and rather salty. He is known as being of large dimension.

THE MALE G-SPOT

The prostate gland is often referred to as the male equivalent of the woman's G-spot, because of its sexual sensitivity and the similarity of its sexual response. Surprisingly, most Western heterosexual men have never considered the prostate as part of their sexual apparatus.

A man's prostate is a muscular gland about the size and shape of a walnut. It is located at the root of the lingam, inside the body, and is part of his urinary and reproductive system. It also contributes to the pleasure felt during arousal and ejaculation. The prostate is just below the bladder and its two semicircular lobes (one on the left, one on the right) encircle the urethra. The urethra is the tube that carries urine

The external parts of a man's genitalia are his penis and his scrotum, which contains his testicles, epididymis, and vas deferens. Internally, the main genital organs include the prostate gland and the seminal vesicles.

from the bladder and down through the lingam. One side of the prostate can be felt manually through the wall of the anus facing the penis. A physician will do this during a prostate examination.

The prostate gland has three functions. Because it surrounds the urethra, its muscle fibers can squeeze the urethra slightly and help control the flow of urine. Its second function is the production of fluids that are added to the seminal fluid (semen). The prostate gland is made up of thousands of tiny, fluid-producing glands, which are interspersed within its blood vessels and muscular framework.

When the penis is stimulated, the prostate swells with secretions, and it is estimated that 80 percent of the fluid released during ejaculation comes from the prostate gland. Sperm travels from the testicles upward through the tube called the vas deferens and back down through the prostate gland where it mixes with prostate fluid.

The prostate drains its ejaculatory fluid from its tiny glands into larger tubes or ducts, which then drain into the urethra. Above the prostate gland are the two seminal vesicles which store sperm and ejaculatory fluid. These vesicles are considered to be an extension of the prostate gland.

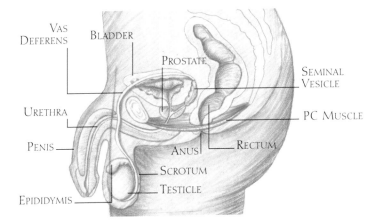

VAS DEFERENS — BLADDER — PROSTATE — SEMINAL VESICLE — PC MUSCLE — URETHRA — PENIS — ANUS — RECTUM — SCROTUM — TESTICLE — EPIDIDYMIS

The third function of the prostate is semen ejaculation. During ejaculation, the muscular sphincter at the base of the bladder tightens and closes, preventing urine from passing down the urethra. Then the prostate undergoes a rapid series of contractions. These contractions squeeze the secretions from the prostate, which shrinks and returns to its normal size. The ejaculate, now containing both sperm and seminal fluid, passes from the ejaculatory ducts into the urethra, then it flows along the urethra and spurts out through the end of the lingam.

Each time the prostate contracts and relaxes, it draws sperm from the seminal vesicles. It is possible for a man to experience up to twenty-one contractions. With the pumping of the prostate preceding ejaculation, the man feels the pleasurable sensations that he generally associates with orgasm.

PROSTATE MASSAGE

Massage of the prostate is sometimes perceived as unpleasant, particularly when part of a medical examination. However, when the prostate is massaged during masturbation or as part of a sexual encounter, most men find the sensation extremely pleasurable. It is easier to feel your prostate when you have an erection.

To give yourself a prostate massage, lie on your back with your knees up and your feet flat on the bed, and use the following simple techniques:

- Use saliva, a water-based lubricant, or one made with natural ingredients to facilitate finger or thumb insertion.
- Massage your prostate by simply inserting your finger into your anus and reaching back and up toward the navel until you feel the prostate. It feels like a firm mass about the size of a walnut and is normally rubbery, pliable, and smooth. Simply rub back and forth on the prostate, applying as much pressure as you can without causing pain.
- Alternatively, gently insert your thumb into your rectum and press against the anterior (front) rectal wall, massaging down toward the anus.
- A rhythmic, pulsing pressure applied every now and then is not only pleasurable but also a reliable way to prolong arousal and delay ejaculation. Apply the pressure via your anus or through your perineum (the area between your scrotum and anus).

If your lover is willing to do it for you, your prostate massage will be made even more pleasurable.

PROSTATE LOVEPLAY

Many men and women have a very negative attitude to anal touching, which is unfortunate because they're missing out on an important source of sexual pleasure. The prostate gland is rich in sensitive nerve endings, so it becomes aroused very easily and stimulating it during lovemaking often results in an intense orgasm. But feelings of vulnerability are very common with any kind of anal stimulation, so to explore this erogenous zone completely with your lover you need to feel relaxed, trusting, and comfortable as well as experimental and playful!

For both men and women, opening up to a gentle finger in the anus can lead to a wonderful new realm of sexual responsiveness. And when a man's prostate is stimulated it can intensify and prolong his orgasm. Combining prostate stimulation with lingam stimulation during masturbation or lovemaking may lead to new orgasm experiences for you.

Some men like to have their prostates touched only when they are fully aroused; others feel that having their prostates stimulated increases erections and leads to the best orgasms. And there are some men who do not even need to have their lingams stimulated, because the feeling that comes from the prostate's manipulation is enough to trigger an orgasm.

If you and your lover want to introduce prostate stimulation into your loveplay, here's how to do it:

- To explore your prostate during sex, your lover should slowly and gently insert a well-lubricated finger (making sure nails are trimmed and clean!) into your anus. Although it may feel strange initially, give it a moment because it will soon feel incredible. It's not necessary to insert the entire finger because it's the outermost third of the rectum that is the most sensitive for the prostate.
- To help relax the surrounding area, your lover should slowly move her finger in and out. When both of you are feeling comfortable with the finger fully inside, your lover should curl her finger and do a beckoning "come here" movement with it so that the tip of her finger taps on your prostate. Some men are able to orgasm from this form of stimulation alone, while others desire this form of stimulation combined with oral sex.
- If your lover is willing, let her stimulate your anus by rubbing it on the outside while giving you oral sex. For many men, this simultaneous lingam and anal stimulation is an incredibly arousing feeling!

Please remember that good hygiene is an essential part of safe lovemaking. If you insert a finger or anything else into the rectum, never bring it in contact with other parts of the body without first washing it with soap and water.

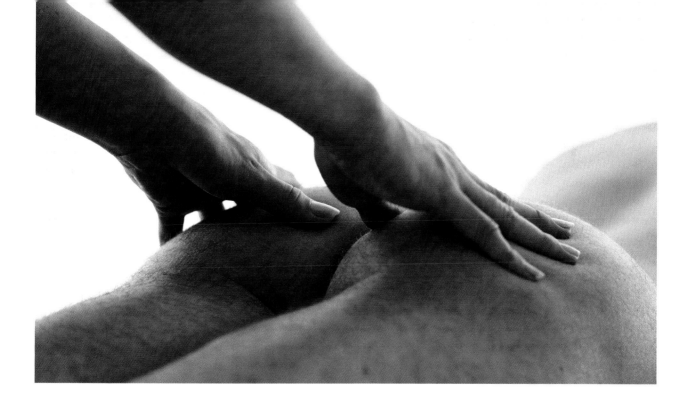

PROSTATE CARE

There is nothing "dirty" about enjoying anal stimulation, but your body does need to be cared for and looked after. You can help prevent disease and infections by taking proper care of your entire body including your anus and your prostate.

When you get aroused, your prostate naturally enlarges slightly. To help control ejaculation and to relieve pressure on your prostate, practice contracting your PC (pubococcygeus) muscle around your prostate before and after self-pleasuring or lovemaking. Your PC muscle (see page 32) is the one you use to control the flow of urine when you pee. You can also massage your perineum, testicles, and tailbone to help relieve pressure and disperse the built-up sexual energy when practicing withholding ejaculation (see page 38).

If your prostate feels enlarged or hard, or you can feel a hard lump on it, these are indications that it has undergone a change, and if it is swollen, sore, and soft it may be infected. If you or your lover detect any such changes to your prostate, you should seek proper medical advice without delay.

To explore the erogenous potential of your prostate, you need to feel comfortable, experimental, and playful!

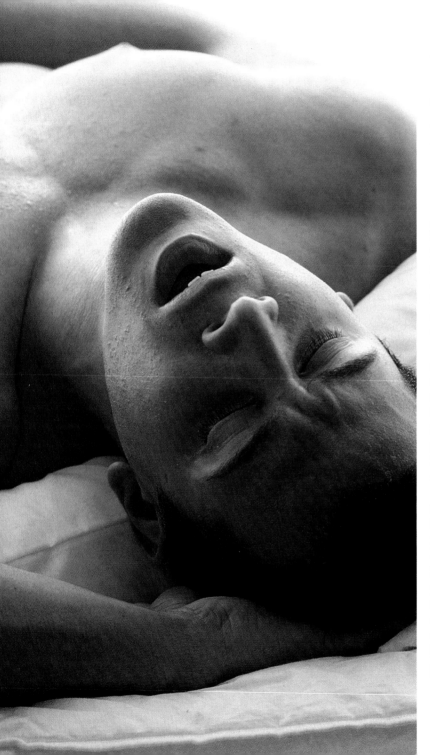

ORGASM AND EJACULATION

Many people find it surprising that a man can have an orgasm without ejaculating, because they have learned to associate the male orgasm with the moment of ejaculation. But orgasm and ejaculation are actually two distinctly different bodily responses, and men can experience the bliss of orgasm both with and without ejaculation.

By breaking the link between orgasm and ejaculation (and the necessary recovery period that follows it), men can learn to have multiple orgasms, just like women. And by learning to refrain from ejaculation they will be able to prolong lovemaking, which will create increased pleasure for both themselves and their partners.

Physiologically, the male orgasm is the set of contractions and pulsations that a man feels in his lingam and prostate when he reaches a sexual climax. It is accompanied by increased heart rate, breathing rate, and blood pressure, and results in a sudden release of tension. Aside from these effects, an orgasm is also the peak experience of sex—whether masturbation or lovemaking—and one of the most pleasurable of all physical experiences.

Ejaculation is the experience of a pleasurable, involuntary muscle spasm that lasts only a few seconds—a reflex that occurs at the base of the spine and results in the ejection of semen and then the loss of the erection. Ejaculation delayed is pleasure magnified. Learning new skills allows lovers to excite and tease their partners to the edge of their precipices, pull them back from the brink, then entice them forward again. Repeatedly and carefully practiced, these skills can lift lovers from peak to peak, each more intense than the last, until they explode into ecstasy.

A woman in ecstasy and surrendered to love is one of nature's most beautiful visions—one that not only boosts her lover's sexual confidence but is also one of the most powerful aphrodisiacs available. By learning to control his ejaculation and to experience the pleasure of multiple orgasms, a man can find enhanced intimacy and love, longer-lasting attraction and passion for his beloved, and levels of ecstasy he never dreamed possible.

WHEN TO EJACULATE

Most men feel tired and drained after ejaculating, because their bodies are then working to replenish the loss of fluids. In Taoist sexology, it is said that when a man ejaculates he is depleting his essence, his *chi* energy. Each time you have an orgasm without ejaculating, you draw more energy into your body. So when you do eventually ejaculate, you still have energy in reserve.

The Taoists recommended that each man ejaculate according to his own physical condition, taking into account his age, his health, and the circumstances of his life. So when you need to conserve more energy, for example during winter months, or if you are unwell, or working hard, you may choose to ejaculate less frequently. On the other hand, if you are on vacation or your partner is trying to conceive, you will probably choose to ejaculate more frequently.

"There is a saying that a man whose Lingam is very long will always be poor. One whose Lingam is very thick will always be in distress. A man who has a thin and lean one will be lucky, and a person whose Lingam is short may well become a king."

ANANGA RANGA

Always remember that you are making love with yourself and with your lover, focusing on "being" with each other and on the exchange of healing love. If you do lose control and feel yourself going past the point of no return, just let go and enjoy it!

THE MULTI-ORGASMIC MALE

It is entirely possible to become multi-orgasmic, just as it is to become a more skillful lover. What it requires is that you learn to understand and master your own arousal process. Allow yourself time to experiment with arousal, erection, and ejaculation—what you discover may surprise you and will certainly delight you.

I recommend starting your "research" through masturbation. This form of self-love enables you to become aware of what is happening within you during sexual arousal. For example, sexual energy expands the emotions you are feeling. So if you focus on loving yourself as you become aroused, your expanding sexual energy will increase your love and will make it much easier to control your ejaculation. Don't hurry the process; the longer you are able to make love with yourself and prolong ejaculation, the faster you will learn to become multi-orgasmic.

THE ESSENTIAL TECHNIQUES

When you have become aware of what happens within you, then you can begin to take control of your ejaculation by using your PC muscle and breathing slowly and deeply (see page 40). These are the two most important techniques for becoming multi-orgasmic.

I recommend that you start off by practicing these alone while masturbating, because this allows you to focus on yourself without having to think about your lover's arousal. It also gives you the opportunity to love yourself physically, and to remain in that loving space rather than using your mind to distract yourself, which takes you out of the moment and leaves you not totally present in the act of love.

SOME PRACTICAL POINTS

- Always urinate before self-pleasuring or lovemaking. A full bladder will make you feel like you need to ejaculate, and make it more difficult for you to withhold ejaculation.
- Use a lubricant to increase your sensations; try your own saliva, or almond or olive oil.
- Give yourself 20 minutes or so, depending on your mood and the moment, to approach orgasm at least three times.
- Notice what is happening in your body as you approach orgasm. How is your breathing? Are you holding your breath? Which muscles are tensing? Has your heart rate speeded up? Is your mouth open or closed? Be aware of the tendency to rush to a climax—relax and try to resist it.

Other techniques to help decrease the urge to ejaculate are pressing the head or base of your lingam with your thumb and finger, or reaching between your legs and pressing on your perineum. Alternatively, combine PC muscle contraction with taking quick shallow breaths, or with taking a deep breath then holding your breath for a few seconds. These methods may also help to disperse the built-up energy.

When you are at the stage of being able to peak without ejaculating, stop and enjoy the sensations. You may feel peaceful and/or energized. Be aware of how sexual energy manifests itself in your body; perhaps as a tingling or pricking sensation rising upward from your genitals. This self-knowledge is the beginning of transforming your genital orgasms into whole-body orgasms.

Be patient with yourself, because it may take a few sessions before you are able to control your ejaculatory orgasm. If you have successfully managed to withhold ejaculation, you may feel a build-up of pressure in your genital area. This is a result of increased blood flow and sexual energy. If the pressure is uncomfortable, simply ejaculate, or breathe deeply and gently massage your perineum, prostate, and testicles. This will help to you absorb the energy, and circulate it out of your genitals and to the rest of your body.

One last, very important point. Many people think that distraction is an essential aid to becoming multi-orgasmic. This is completely erroneous. When a man makes love, his thoughts must be on lovemaking and feeling love.

Desensitizing yourself or distracting yourself with trivia may help to delay ejaculation, but to become multi-orgasmic you have to increase your sexual sensitivity and focus more directly on your sexual arousal.

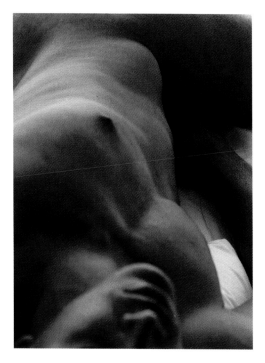

While you masturbate, concentrate on the pleasures that accompany mild arousal and the feelings that occur just before the inevitability of ejaculation. Pay attention, too, to the other changes that for you signal sexual excitation and impending orgasm.

BREATH CONTROL

Learning to control your breathing is an important first step to becoming multi-orgasmic. Your breathing is directly connected to your heart rate: when you breathe quickly your heart rate increases; when you breathe slowly your heart rate decreases. When you are close to ejaculating, the ability to breathe deeply and to slow down your heart rate will be essential. By learning to slow down your breathing, you will learn to control your arousal rate and to experience your orgasms without rushing into ejaculation.

EXERCISING THE PC MUSCLE

The PC or pubococcygeus muscle is actually a group of muscles that run from your pubic bone, in the front of your body, to your tailbone in the back. It is this muscle that you use to stop yourself from urinating or to push out the last few drops of urine. You can feel it behind your testicles and in front of your anus at your perineum. If you strengthen this muscle you will get stronger erections, stronger orgasms, and improved ejaculatory control, which is essential to becoming multi-orgasmic.

The simplest way to strengthen your PC muscle is to squeeze it the next time you urinate. If you have a fairly strong PC muscle, you will be able to stop and start the flow of urine midstream. If

not, practice squeezing the muscle. Begin gradually as the muscle may get a little sore at first. Some men find standing on their toes and clenching their teeth intensifies the practice.

Squeezing and relaxing the muscle may be done anywhere, while driving or watching television, for example, and in any position—sitting, standing, or lying down. Practice using your breath too; breathe in as you contract the muscle and exhale as you relax the muscle.

MAINTAINING ORGASM

With practice, you can learn to keep yourself at an orgasmic level without ejaculating. During intercourse, exhale slowly while thrusting in and inhale slowly while withdrawing. When you do this in a relaxed manner, it creates a steady rhythm that heightens pleasure, helps to relax you, and prevents early ejaculation.

As you approach ejaculation, thrust and withdraw more slowly and change the technique. During withdrawal, inhale and tighten your anus; this causes the head of your lingam to enlarge.

Withdrawing this enlarged lingam head massages the walls of your partner's yoni and provides her with indescribable pleasure. When you thrust, relax and exhale. This technique allows you to maintain an orgasmic level, without ejaculation, for as long as you desire, uniting your mind and your body to create an erotic explosion of sexual energy and pleasure.

Your Lover's Part

The success of all of these techniques depends on the sympathetic help of your lover and whether she assists you to gain control over your ejaculation. Both of you will have to recognize the signs of your heightened arousal, which will include a rapid increase in heart rate, faster breathing, tensing of your muscles, and perhaps jaw tightening or gritting of your teeth.

The speed and depth of your thrusting will also increase. When you reach a high level of arousal near ejaculation, your lover needs to encourage you to make your thrusts shallow and slow. This will have the effect of increasing her stimulation while, hopefully, reducing yours. Alternatively, withdraw completely and rest for a moment before continuing.

Your instinct will be to move toward ejaculation so both of you need to be careful, watching the signs of arousal and stopping or slowing down and changing stimulation when you get too close to release. So, as your lover senses your level of arousal, she needs you to change rhythm and stroke. She has to encourage you to relax and help you with control, while you breathe deeply and practice muscular contractions of your anus and PC muscle. It's important for both of you to remember that ejaculation is not the goal!

Until you have learned the greater pleasures of controlled and extended intercourse, you will push for ejaculation. Your lover must be selfless and loving, and encourage and support you in resisting this urge. And you need to recognize that the experience will ultimately lead to the possibility of extreme levels of ecstatic pleasure for both of you.

It does take time, energy, and a desire to succeed for these practices to be fully effective. If you lose control at first, which is likely in the beginning, it is not a disaster. Just do it again. Be kind to yourselves, enjoy the process of the new experience and be patient and loving with one another.

THE VARIOUS TYPES OF THRUST AS DESCRIBED IN THE *T'UNG HASÜAN TZU*

Deep and shallow, slow and swift, direct and slanting, thrusts are by no means all uniform and each has its own distinctive effect and characteristics. A slow thrust should resemble the jerking movement of a carp toying with a hook; a swift thrust that of the flight of the birds against the wind. Inserting and withdrawing, moving upward and downward, from left to right, interspaced at intervals or in quick succession, and all these should be coordinated. One should apply each at the most suitable time and not always stubbornly cling to only one style alone for reason of one's own laziness or convenience.

1 Strike out to the left and right as a brave warrior trying to break up the enemy ranks.
2 Move up and down as a wild horse bucking through a stream.
3 Pull out and push in as a group of seagulls playing on the waves.
4 Use deep thrusts and shallow teasing strokes, alternating swiftly as a sparrow picking the leftovers of rice in a mortar.
5 Make deep and shallow strokes in steady succession as a huge stone sinking into the sea.
6 Push in slowly as a snake entering a hole to hibernate.
7 Thrust swiftly as a frightened rat rushes into a hole.
8 Poise, then strike like an eagle catching an elusive hare.
9 Rise and then plunge low like a huge sailing boat braving the gale.

LOVING THRUSTS

When lovers are genuinely attracted to one another and know each other's bodies intimately, their lovemaking can be like a beautiful, choreographed dance. But if your lingam always moves in and out of her yoni the same way, your lovemaking can easily become tedious and dull.

Learning how to vary the rhythm and depth of your thrusts will help make your loving last longer, and add variety so you both experience more pleasure. Try different thrusts at different speeds, intensities, and depths (see left). The variations will help you to keep your lingam strong and erect, and make it easier for you to control ejaculation.

ERECTION PROBLEMS

It is not uncommon for a man to feel ashamed and embarrassed if his lingam fails him and he is unable to achieve erection. Men and women need to recognize that it's just a normal part of male sexuality and it can happen to men of any age. Some are convinced that it means the end of their sex lives, but usually it's just an isolated moment or a passing phase. Most men find that it is easy to remedy with masturbation, breathing exercises, and PC muscle contractions, or using a light touch with an electric massager.

Although some physical ailments (and some forms of medication) may cause erection problems, the cause is most often psychological. Many men don't understand that the occasional failure to get an erection is a common and natural occurrence, often the result of factors such as stress, fatigue, or alcohol. Because of this lack of understanding, a single failure to get an erection can sometimes trigger a deep-seated fear of permanent impotence—a fear that is one of the main factors in many cases of long-term impotence.

Impotence normally becomes a major problem when the man *feels* that it is a major problem. When a man puts unnecessary pressure upon himself to perform, he usually becomes more frustrated and less able to. If impotence is a problem between you and your lover, there are many techniques that you can try before you resort to visiting a doctor or a sex therapist.

RELEARNING HOW TO STIMULATE

As a man gets older, he generally needs more stimulation to become erect. Some men find that the only thing that will give them an erection is oral stimulation, while others need almost constant manual stimulation to achieve one. If manual stimulation is what you need, avoid pulling too vigorously on the lingam, or squeezing it too tightly, because that may reduce the erection.

COMBATING IMPOTENCE

If you are having erection problems, it's vital that you to talk to your lover and express your concerns. This can help to ease the tension and clear the way for you to start overcoming the problem together. The next step is to ensure that you are comfortable. If you are under a lot of stress, you may have difficulty achieving erection. If you feel relaxed, it will be easier for you to become erect. Always remember that you don't need a hard lingam to be sexual.

There are many ways to be a great lover—kissing and caressing, oral loving,

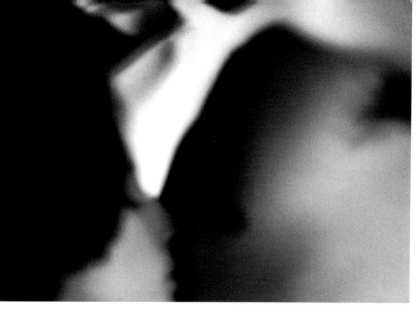

massage, using a dildo for vaginal and/or anal penetration, using a vibrator, fantasy role-playing, and mutual masturbation. The important thing is to relax, enjoy yourself, and not worry about your erection—concentrate on your lover's erotic stimulation. The more arousing attention you give your lover, the greater the possibility for your own arousal. Her excitement might be enough to give you an erection, but if it doesn't, you can still make love to her by using the soft entry method.

THE SOFT ENTRY METHOD

The soft entry method ("enter soft, exit hard") is a way of entering your lover without an erection but with a little help from your fingers. It is worth practicing even if you don't have any erection problems, because no man can be sure

of being able to get an erection every time he wants one. Soft entry can be an exciting new experience for a woman if it is well managed, and it can also be helpful when you want to make love again soon after ejaculating.

The most convenient positions for soft entry are side-by-side facing one another or man-on-top. In these positions you have as much freedom to move as possible.

You begin by fondling and caressing one another. Spend time arousing your lover so she becomes well lubricated with her own fluids, or apply plenty of water-based lubricant to the head and shaft of your lingam (or to the condom, if you're using one). Then use your thumb and index finger to form a ring around the base of your lingam, and squeeze firmly to make the upper part of it at least semi-rigid. You should now be able to maneuver your lingam into her yoni, and—still squeezing—you can carefully start to thrust. Once you begin thrusting, your erection might well firm up enough for you to let go of the base of your lingam. Your lover can help, too, by stroking your testicles and pressing on your perineum, or by fingering your anus if you enjoy anal stimulation.

Soft entry is not guaranteed to work every time, or for every man. But for those who learn to use it, it offers a very good chance of success.

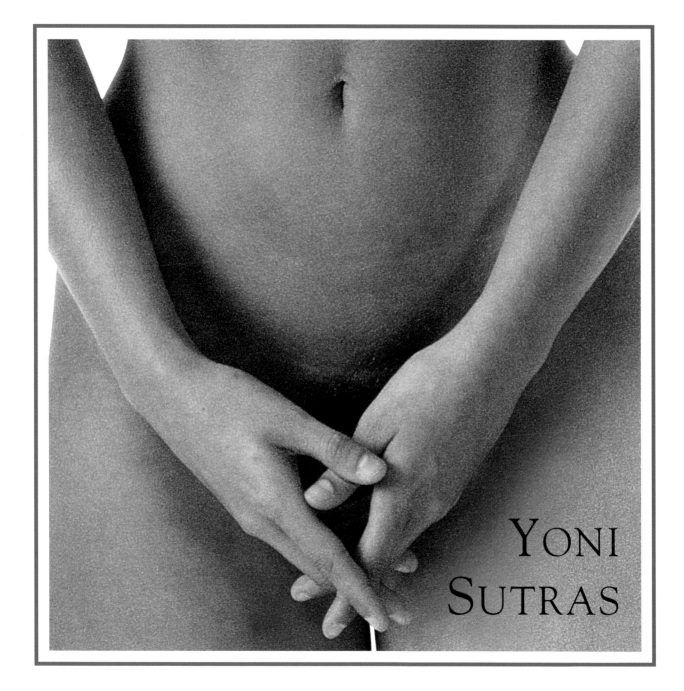

YONI
SUTRAS

THE YONI

"The term yoni heralds from a culture and religion in which women have long been regarded and honored as the embodiment of divine female energy—the energy known as Shakti—and where the female genitals are seen as a sacred symbol of the Great Goddess."

RUFUS C. CAMPHAUSEN

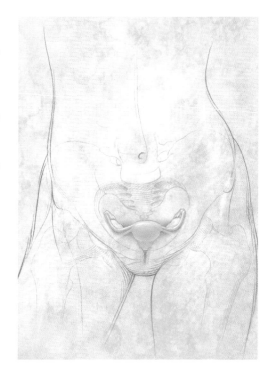

The word "yoni" is a sanskrit term that translates as "womb," "origin," and "source," and more specifically as "vulva." The yoni is the source of all life, pleasure, and beauty, and it incorporates the generative principle. In Indian tradition, the yoni is viewed as the entrance to the original sacred shrine, and it is used in the worship of Shakti, the female creative force and the embodiment of receptivity. The *padma* or lotus is a frequent symbol for the female genitalia in the East. In the West, the yoni is most often symbolized by the rose.

In describing the vulva and vagina, I prefer to use the word "yoni" because it is more poetic and less clinical. It also emphasizes the extraordinary beauty of this part of the female body and the reverence owed to it.

The yoni is regarded as the source of all life, pleasure, and beauty, and said to incorporate the generative principle.

Yoni Essentials

The outer parts of the female genitalia consist of the mons veneris, the labia (vaginal lips), and the clitoris. The mons veneris, or mound of Venus, is a layer of fat that covers the pubic bone, and it divides to form the outer vaginal lips (the labia majora). Inside these are the inner lips (the labia minora), the urethral opening, and the entrance to the vagina. The inner lips join at the top to form the "hood" that protects the highly sensitive head of the clitoris when it is in its unerect state; pull the hood back and you will expose the clitoris.

During sexual arousal, a woman's vaginal lips become swollen and their color deepens. The shaft of her clitoris thickens and shortens and becomes erect, and her vagina lengthens, expands, and excretes a lubricating fluid. At the same time, her breasts swell and her nipples become erect.

If the arousal continues, her clitoris enlarges further, and it seems to disappear. This is because it pulls back against the pubic bone and is covered by the swollen vaginal lips.

During orgasm, a woman's heart rate will more than double, her breathing is more than three times as fast as normal, and the outer third of her vagina (the orgasmic platform) contracts rhythmically, typically from three to 15 times in as many seconds.

THE THREE TYPES OF FEMALE SEX ORGANS ACCORDING TO THE *KAMA SUTRA* AND THE *ANANGA RANGA*

THE DEER

This is a Yoni that does not exceed six finger-breadths (about 5 inches) in depth. Usually a woman with such a Yoni has a soft and girlish body, well proportioned with good breasts and solid hips. She eats moderately and is addicted to the pleasures of lovemaking. Her mind is very active and her Yoni juice has the pleasant perfume of the lotus flower. She is known as being of small dimension.

THE MARE

This is the Yoni that does not exceed nine finger-breadths (about seven inches) in depth. Usually this woman's body is delicate, her breasts and hips are broad, and her umbilical region is raised. She has well-proportioned hands and feet, a long neck, and a retreating forehead. Her throat, eyes, and mouth are broad, and her eyes are very beautiful. She is very versatile, affectionate, and graceful, and likes good living and lots of rest. She does not easily come to her climax and her love juice is perfumed like the lotus. She is known as being of middle dimension.

THE ELEPHANT

This is the Yoni that is about twelve finger-breadths (about 10 inches) in depth. This woman usually has large breasts, a broad face, and fairly short limbs. She is gluttonous and eats noisily; her voice is hard and harsh. Such a woman is never easily satisfied, but her love juice is very abundant and smells rather like the secretions of an elephant in rut. She is known as being of large dimension.

"The Valley spirit never dies. It is named the mysterious female. And the doorway of the mysterious female is the base from which heaven and earth sprang. It is there within us all the while; draw upon it as you will, it never runs dry."

TAO TE CHING

THE CLITORIS

The word "clitoris" comes from the Greek word *kleitoris,* meaning "the female genitals." Other words for the clitoris include the Chinese terms that translate as "golden tongue," "seat of pleasure," and "jade terrace."

A good understanding of the clitoris is essential to the sexual health and emotional happiness of women. Yet in the past, the majority of sex books and manuals paid very little attention to it other than to describe it as a pea-size organ whose sole purpose is that of providing pleasure.

It is true that a woman can experience sexual pleasure and/or orgasm without knowing anything about her anatomy, or indeed, without touching any part of it. The more informed you become about your physical self, the greater potential for pleasure you have.

Knowing that there is so much more to the clitoris than just the glans may lead you to the path of discovery about your sexual potential, as well as increasing your own capacity for pleasure. This knowledge is important, especially for women, not least because of the powerful impact that this small organ has on the female orgasm.

The clitoris is the key to sexual pleasure for the majority of women. Only women are endowed with an organ that has just one purpose: pleasure. Its ability to receive and transmit sensations of touch, pressure, and vibration is unsurpassed. It is a source of immense pleasure for women and an essential part of the process that leads to orgasm.

There are many possible variations in the size and appearance of the clitoris. But it is much more than the exposed pea-size organ or "bud" that you can see. It is actually part of a much larger organ. All parts of the clitoris function together to provide sexual pleasure and orgasm, but the clitoris is certainly more than the sum of its parts.

The clitoris holds between 6,000 and 8,000 sensory nerve endings, more than any other structure in the human body—male or female—and four times as many as the glans of the lingam. In total, the clitoris is about four inches long, and when the tip is stimulated by fingers, tongue, toys, or lingam, the entire thing engorges and becomes firm and sensitive.

Rebecca Chalker, in her book *The Clitoral Truth*, points out that the clitoris and lingam were considered equivalent in most respects for more than 2,500 years. But from the 18th century, this knowledge was gradually repressed and forgotten and the definition of the clitoris shrank from an extensive organ system to a teeny pea-size bump. Her theory is that this was possibly, or even certainly, the result of a "male-centered, heterosexual model of sexuality."

It was not until 1966, when feminist psychiatrist Mary Jane Sherfe published an article about female sexuality, that the clitoris began to take shape again, so to speak. The process of precisely defining the anatomy of the entire clitoris was completed in 1981 by researchers from the Federation of Feminist Women's Health Centers, who identified 18 individual parts.

Clitoral Anatomy

The clitoris consists of a rounded tip (the glans or crown), attached to a longer part (the shaft). The shaft has two "arms" (called crura) that stretch backward into the woman's body, under the skin on either side above the vaginal opening. Nerves controlling clitoral muscle contractions travel alongside the

walls of the vagina, the bladder, and the urethra, passing along the sensations produced in any part of the region. Usually only the glans of the clitoris is visible, because the labia minora meet over the shaft of the clitoris to form a hood called the prepuce.

Like the lingam, both the glans and the shaft of the clitoris contain spongy, erectile tissue. This tissue fills with

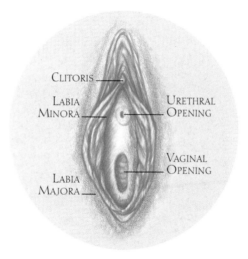

CLITORIS

LABIA MINORA

URETHRAL OPENING

VAGINAL OPENING

LABIA MAJORA

The inner lips of the vagina join at the top to form the protective hood of the clitoris. Effectiuve stimulation of the clitoris is the key to sexual pleasure for the majority of women.

blood during arousal, causing the clitoris to nearly double in size. However, there is no evidence that a larger clitoris means more intense sexual arousal.

The nerve endings in the clitoris make the organ highly sensitive to any kind of touch or pressure. Stimulating a woman physically and mentally can cause the clitoris, labia, and the surrounding area to become swollen with blood, much like an erect lingam.

As a woman continues to become more aroused, the clitoris becomes less visible as the tissues in the clitoral hood swell, covering it and protecting it from direct contact, which can be too intense for many women. After orgasm (or after the stimulation stops), the blood drains from the clitoral area and it returns to its normal size.

The clitoris is becoming a very fashionable body part to adorn with piercings. Some women like the esthetics of a clitoral ring or bar; others do it for spiritual or personal reasons. The most common reason for piercing the clitoris or clitoral hood is for increased orgasm intensity. Not all women report better orgasms as a result of genital piercing, but those that do so have some great stories to tell.

There's nothing physiologically wrong with piercing your genitals (or any other part of your anatomy), just make sure the piercing is performed in clean, hygienic conditions. Also be aware that clitoral piercings can be more painful and take much longer to heal than other body piercings.

As estrogen production in women declines as they get older, a number of changes occur that influence their sexual responses. For some women these changes may include decreased clitoral sensitivity, and the clitoris may change in size with age.

EXPLORING THE YONI

It is extraordinary, to me, that here we are in the twenty-first century and there continues to be a sense of shame and guilt concerned with sex and sexuality, and the functions of the human body.

As a woman, and one in her early forties, I have been aware for some time (as a result of the contact and conversations I have had with other women) of the importance to women of reclaiming our goddesshood. This involves taking responsibility for our own pleasure and our understanding and awareness of our own bodies and seats of pleasure. Almost all of us are affected by socially imposed negative attitudes toward sex and different areas of the human body. Repression results in an inability to touch and explore our own bodies for sexual pleasure. And, all too often, unnecessary suffering is caused by a simple lack of information.

After reading Betty Dodson's *Sex for One*, I realized I had no idea what my genitalia really looked like and how mine compared to other women's. All I knew, and only because I asked my lovers, was that all women are totally unique. As with the rest of nature, there are no two of anything exactly alike.

Before we go farther and deeper, I urge you at this point to take the time to have a good look at your own yoni. You need to become aware that the origin of the energy for sexual pleasures lies inside your own body. We tend to devote a lot of time and energy to things we can see, like our faces and our hair, and we neglect the unseen parts of ourselves.

I really encourage you to do this as an exercise on your own initially, and then to share the experience and your findings with your lover. Find a comfortable sitting position where there is good lighting; you may want soft pillows or cushions to support yourself. You will need a mirror in which to look at your yoni, preferably one that you can prop up to leave your hands free. You may even want to use an instant picture camera to photograph yourself, so that you can see yourself as you never have before.

Explore your yoni with the same attention and interest that you devote to your face and other areas of your body. Take a few minutes to identify the different parts of your yoni—the clitoris, labia, and urethra—and your perineum and anus. Pull your outer lips apart and look inside. Pay attention to your inner lips. Notice their size and shape, the different colors and textures, and where it is moist or dry.

Examine your clitoris and the hood that protects it. See if you are able to move the hood up and down along the shaft of the clitoris. What color is your clitoris? What size and shape is it? Touch and caress it and explore the variety of sensations. Put a finger either side of your clitoral shaft and move them back and forth. Notice if your clitoris swells and changes color with the stimulation.

Open your lips with your fingers, and explore the inside of your yoni with your fingers. Do this first when you are in an unaroused state and then again when you are aroused. Take a few deep breaths to relax and gently press around the inside of your yoni, circling your fingers and noting the different sensations and feelings. Where is it smooth and where do you feel ridges? Contract your pelvic floor muscles and notice the grip on your finger or fingers.

If you begin to become aroused, notice how your yoni swells and moistens with pleasure. Then withdraw your finger or fingers and look at your wetness. Does it have a color or particular consistency? What does it smell and taste like? This varies considerably with each woman, day to day, and at different times of the monthly cycle. Become familiar with what your yoni looks like, smells like, and tastes like, and learn to love and appreciate ALL of you.

THE G-SPOT—THE JEWEL IN THE LOTUS

"How delicious an instrument is woman, when artfully played upon; how capable is she of producing the most exquisite harmonies, of executing the most complicated variations of love, and of giving the most Divine of erotic pleasures."

ANANGA RANGA

The Gräfenberg spot or "G-spot" (named for the man who "discovered" it) is a hypersensitive area inside the vagina. The area of the G-spot is known also as the urethral sponge, an area of spongy tissue that also contains clusters of nerve endings, blood vessels, and paraurethral glands and ducts. It covers the female urethra (urinary tube) on all sides. During sexual stimulation by finger pressure, or certain positions and movements of the lingam, the "sponge" can become engorged with blood. It swells, becomes distinguishable to the touch, and has the ability to ejaculate an orgasmic fluid, referred to by the Chinese as "moon flower medicine" or "moon flower water."

Every woman has this area or region in her vagina, but each woman experiences it differently. Its sensitivity varies from woman to woman and depends upon a wide variety of psychological and physical factors. When a woman becomes sexually aroused, the area swells and so becomes more sensitive to stimulation, which for some women leads to a deeper and more satisfying orgasm and even ejaculation. It is also not uncommon, when the G-spot is massaged, to feel as though you need to urinate, but if you continue stimulation you will experience the transition to sexual arousal. While the G-spot is the most famous, there are other sensitive spots inside the yoni that are unique to each woman.

LOCATING THE G-SPOT

The G-spot can be felt along the front wall of the vagina, on the belly side, approximately two inches from the entrance of the yoni. It is a well-hidden spot, deep within the vaginal wall and about the size of a bean, though the size and exact location vary from woman to woman. And it can be difficult to locate it if you are not sexually aroused. The best position to be in to locate it yourself is either to squat or to lie down with your legs in the air. Then insert your middle finger into your yoni and gently press and probe with it to seek out your G-spot.

LOVEMAKING AND THE G-SPOT
The most effective positions are those where the woman can control the depth of the man's penetration and guide his lingam to stimulate her G-spot. Rear-entry positions work well, with both lovers on their knees (doggie style) or with the woman lying on her belly with a pillow under her waist and the man behind on top. These positions allow the man to move up over his partner in a more vertical position, and to use shallower thrusts to stimulate her G-spot.

Also good is if she lies on her back with her legs raised and her feet on his shoulders,

or if he lies on his back and she sits on top facing his feet. In the latter pose she can, if she is supple enough, lean back on her hands toward his chest.

Another position for G-spot stimulation is where the woman lies on her back, knees bent into her chest, with her ankles crossed and resting against the man's upper body. He is on his knees facing her with his hands on her thighs. It is also possible to stimulate the G-spot by using external pressure on the abdomen, slightly above the pubic bone, either with a lover or during self-pleasuring.

To stimulate her G-spot during intercourse, try the cross-legged position (above) or a rear-entry position (left).

THE LOVE MUSCLE

The PC (pubococcygeus) muscle is the most important muscle for increasing, improving, expanding, exploring, and enjoying one's sexuality. The better the health and condition of this muscle, the more enjoyment both men and women will derive from sex. A healthy PC muscle is generally more sensitive to physical stimulation than a weak one, while sometimes a weak muscle may be partially responsible for a woman's failure to reach orgasm during intercourse.

Like any other muscle in the body, the PC—or "love muscle"—can be educated and trained through proper exercise. Strengthening the muscle improves blood flow and circulation to and around the yoni (including the G-spot and perineum), and helps to increase lubrication and sexual energy. The stronger the muscle, the more pleasure you feel and the greater your sexual and orgasmic response.

Exercising and strengthening the PC muscle throughout your life is an important part of maintaining your health and realizing your sexual potential. Childbirth and the process of ageing weakens the muscle, and unless it is exercised regularly its strength will decrease. This is often the reason that women have difficulty holding in urine later in life. PC muscle exercises will also improve vaginal lubrication and are valuable for older, postmenopausal women who may suffer from dryness of the vaginal lining.

LOCATING THE PC MUSCLE

The easiest way to locate the muscle is to practice stopping and starting your stream of urine as you empty your bladder. Contract your PC muscle—the sensation is that of pulling up—and then push down as if you were having a bowel movement. If you notice your stomach, buttocks, and thigh muscles move at the same time, you need to learn to isolate the PC muscle.

Another way to locate the muscle is by putting a finger in your yoni and

Also known as the pelvic floor muscles, the PC muscle is actually a group of muscles at the bottom of your pelvis, extending from the pubic bone to the tailbone. Acting as a muscular sling, it supports all your sexual and reproductive organs as well as your urethra and rectum.

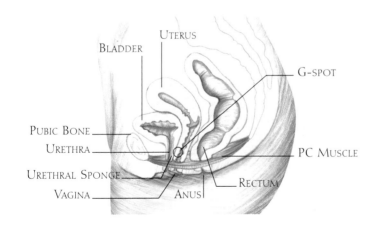

UTERUS

BLADDER

G-SPOT

PUBIC BONE

URETHRA

PC MUSCLE

URETHRAL SPONGE

RECTUM

VAGINA

ANUS

squeezing. The muscle you use is your PC muscle. The contraction feels like you are pulling your yoni up and slightly into your body, and it can be felt in your clitoris, vagina, and anus. Then try inserting two fingers side-by-side as deep as you comfortably can. Spread your fingers apart as if opening a pair of scissors. Now contract your PC muscle to force your fingers to come together. If you find this difficult, you need exercise!

PC Muscle Exercises

Muscle improvement relies on frequent and regular practice. It's a good idea to use a resistive device that gives the muscle something to squeeze against. This could be your lover's lingam, a dildo, or fingers—your own or your lover's. It needs to be something firm but with some give. It is also possible to buy a "barbell" specifically designed for a woman's yoni.

Set aside time for two fifteen-minute sessions a day. Using your resistive device, contract your PC muscle and hold for three seconds, then release and relax for three seconds. If you cannot manage three seconds, do one or two. Eventually, with practice, you should be able to build up gradually to ten seconds, and always relax for the same amount of time between each contraction. Practice a series of ten contractions and releases, and then squeeze and release the muscle as quickly as possible for as long as you can. Like any other muscle that you reintroduce exercise to, it makes sense to start gradually so as not to strain it.

PC muscle exercises without a resistive object are also extremely effective, and you can practice them undetected at any time, anywhere, and in any position. Having said that, some women find the contractions very sexually stimulating, which may then be reflected in their breathing or blushing! When you are familiar with the sensation of contracting and relaxing your PC muscle, you can vary the length of contraction and release and the number of repetitions, and incorporate your breathing into the exercise. Begin by breathing in, contracting the muscle for 5 or 10 seconds then breathing out as you release. Next, repeat the same exercise, but this time reverse the breathing so you exhale as you contract the muscle and inhale as you release it. Then try "fluttering" the muscle, contracting and relaxing it as quickly as possible for as long as you can manage.

It is also useful to practice PC contractions against your lover's lingam during intercourse, and ask if he can feel them. Depending on the state of your muscle, it may take anything from

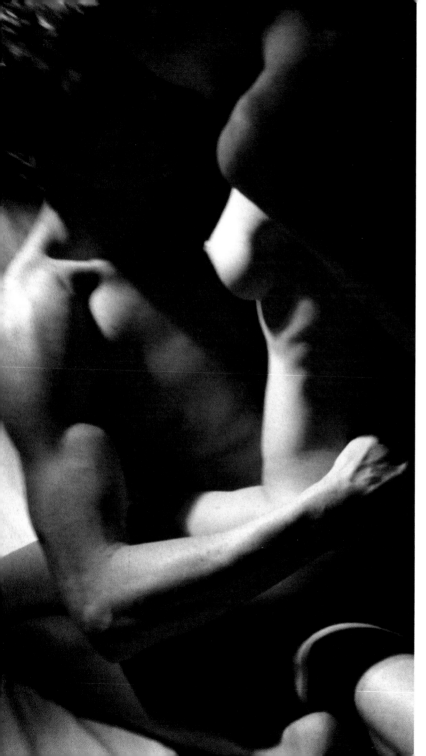

a few days to a few weeks before he will notice—but he will notice! Contracting against his lingam as it withdraws will create a kind of suction of the vaginal walls, increasing stimulation and pleasure for you both.

PC TREASURES

With a developed PC muscle, there are some sensational treats in store for you when self pleasuring using a dildo or during intercourse with your lover.

- As your lover's lingam enters your yoni, contract your muscles rhythmically around the head.
- As he slowly penetrates, contract your PC muscle rhythmically as if you were sucking his lingam into your yoni.
- As he thrusts in and out, relax the muscles when he thrusts and squeeze your PC muscle as he withdraws.
- When you practice the Sets of Nine with your lover (see page 59), tighten your PC muscle as he withdraws during the shallow thrusts, and squeeze continuously as he moves in and out during the deep thrusts.

FEMALE ORGASM

Firstly, there is no one "right" or "normal" way to experience orgasm; there are many ways, and just as we are each unique and individual, so is our experience of orgasm. It is generally accepted that women have the capacity for almost inexhaustible sexual pleasure. Some women experience more than one type of orgasm, some women have multiple orgasms, and some only have orgasms sometimes. Some women have orgasms only with a particular lover, some have them only while self-pleasuring, and some do not think they have orgasms at all. The thing about orgasms is that women experience them differently and with varying intensity.

Orgasms are associated with the stimulation of different genital areas — internal, external, or a combination of both. The clitoris is the most common area of stimulation and pleasure. Women who do experience orgasm do so as a result of direct stimulation of the clitoris by the tongue, fingers, or vibrators, or by the friction created against the lingam in different lovemaking postures.

It is possible that some women are not capable of orgasm, and for them just the experience of physical and emotional closeness with their lovers may be considered the most enjoyable aspect of sex and be more important than orgasm. There are many ecstatic experiences available in life and they are not all associated with sex and orgasm. The most important thing is to be able to enjoy exploring your sexual potential within a loving relationship. While information and education are important too, the pressure to perform or conform will inhibit rather than increase sexual enjoyment.

The first step to becoming orgasmic is to let go of expectation. When there is no goal it allows you to remain fully present in the moment and experience all the sensations as they happen. Unfortunately, we in the West are very goal-oriented. We believe that sex must end with orgasm to be fulfilling and satisfying, and for men, orgasm equals ejaculation. When so much focus is placed on the end, we miss each moment of the journey.

All of us, however, can enhance our pleasure and satisfaction through better understanding, and open ourselves to greater possibilities of sexual and loving ecstasy with or without orgasms. The most important thing is to enjoy the journey of self-discovery—alone or with your lover—without the pressure to achieve or to perform. Experience what you experience in each moment fully and completely. Stay present and remain open and all good things will surely come to you.

ENHANCING AROUSAL

As a first step to achieving orgasm, become familiar with your sexual anatomy and what you find arousing.

• Explore the different areas of your entire body as well as your yoni, internally and externally. Get to know where your body responds to touch, and how it reacts to different types. Use a vibrator or dildo to stimulate

"A woman in orgasm can be described as a blossoming lotus flower. A woman experiencing a complete orgasm all nine levels of orgasm—undergoes nine stages of blossoming until she finally opens up and surrenders herself to the lover who has served her."

STEPHEN CHANG

your G-spot (see page 52); use your PC muscle (see page 54) for rhythmic contractions and releases. If you are able to pleasure yourself, it is much easier to help a lover to pleasure you.

• If you respond well to clitoral stimulation, don't be afraid to stimulate yourself while making love, adjust your position to increase the

stimulation, or show your lover how to touch you there. Simultaneous nipple and clitoral (or clitoral and G-spot) stimulation with hands, mouth, or lingam may help to increase arousal.

• The largest sex organ of both men's and women's bodies is the mind, so it is vital that you believe that you are capable of experiencing intense pleasure. Stimulate your sensual being, by creating the necessary mood and ambience with candles, music, or with whatever else turns you on. Try different locations and particular times of day. Explore and experiment with erotic literature, photographs, or film. And your imagination will always help you to increase your desire and arousal, so use it!

• Be verbally specific about what you like and what feels good, and thank your partner when he does what you want. If you like your clitoris to be rubbed, stroked, or massaged, let your lover know. If you like your lover to whisper in your ear, or you like your lower back tapped or your fingers or toes sucked—whatever it is that turns you on—dare to ask for it.

• If you want lubrication to increase the sensation, use your own or your lover's saliva, or almond or olive oil.

• Using the breath can also be a great help for increasing arousal. Use deep rhythmic breaths, without straining, to open your chest and belly. Making sounds is another effective way of raising sexual energy levels.

- Don't be afraid to touch yourself in front of your lover. If you stimulate yourself, it's not only educational for him, it can also be a great turn-on.
- Teasing is a technique you can use whether you are arousing yourself or you're with a lover. When you reach a point of moderate desire, hold back on the stimulation until it decreases (but don't let it disappear altogether). Then increase stimulation again and back off again. Repeat this, each time slowly increasing the intensity of your pleasure and suspense. If you experience orgasm, your sexual energy will be high, and if stimulation continues, you can maintain your level of arousal and possibly build to another orgasm with the same stimulation-and-holdback method. Your lover may also tease you with his lingam at the entrance to your yoni, moving slowly to penetration and to positions that stimulate the G-spot.

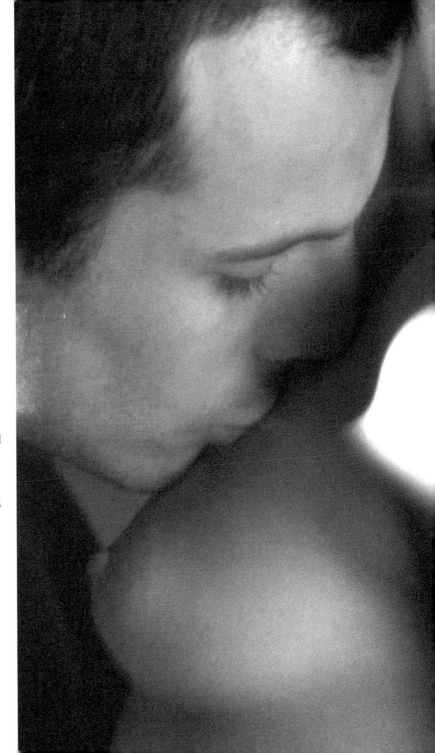

SETS OF NINE

This is an intercourse technique that a man can use during lovemaking to help his beloved to achieve the nine levels of orgasm (see opposite page).

The first Set of Nine consists of nine shallow thrusts and one deep thrust. It heightens pleasure, helps to prevent early ejaculation, and maintains a high level of awareness and concentration—and women find it extremely arousing. The man thrusts slowly, gently, and lovingly. For the first nine strokes, he allows only the head of his lingam to penetrate his lover's yoni; these are the shallow thrusts.

On the deep thrust, he allows the entire length of the lingam to penetrate. Besides its sensory stimulation, this forces air out of the yoni. This creates a partial vacuum within the yoni during the shallow thrusts, making the woman feel first tantalized then satisfied. While thrusting, the man must take care not to withdraw completely.

After nine shallow thrusts and one deep thrust, he follows with:
• eight shallow and two deep thrusts
• seven shallow and three deep thrusts
• six shallow and four deep thrusts
• five shallow and five deep thrusts
• four shallow and six deep thrusts
• three shallow and seven deep thrusts
• two shallow and eight deep thrusts
• one shallow and nine deep thrusts.

The aim is to go through as many Sets of Nine as possible without ejaculating. The best results and the most pleasure are achieved when the pace is slow. When the lingam is nearly withdrawn from the yoni, the yoni will instinctively react by contracting to hold onto it. The yoni's instinctive reaction will heighten the woman's psychological expectation as she awaits repenetration by her lover's lingam.

To increase her pleasure further, the woman will benefit from the conscious effort of contracting and tightening her yoni as her lover withdraws. This contraction results in more friction, more stimulation, and more pleasure. Men often find this amount of stimulation overwhelming at first, so it is important to vary the number of sets and the pace according to individual ability. For the man, the rhythm and the even stimulation of the head and shaft of the lingam helps to delay ejaculation. This prolongs intercourse and creates an even more powerful experience of orgasm for him.

THE NINE LEVELS OF FEMALE ORGASM

ACCORDING TO *THE TAO OF SEXOLOGY*, THE NINE LEVELS OF FEMALE ORGASM ARE:

LEVEL	ENERGIZED ORGANS	THE WOMAN'S RESPONSE
1	LUNGS	She sighs and her breath is short or she breathes heavily and salivates
2	HEART	She extends her tongue while kissing the man and her heart speeds up
3	SPLEEN, PANCREAS, AND STOMACH	Her muscles become activated and she grasps and holds him tightly; her saliva increases so much she may have a cold tongue (sure sign)
4	KIDNEYS AND BLADDER	Vaginal spasms start and fluids begin to flow
5	BONES	Her joints loosen; she bites the man or she curls up and holds him tight
6	LIVER AND NERVES	She undulates and gyrates, wrapping her arms and legs around him, and she may start to bite
7	BLOOD	Her blood is "boiling." She perspires heavily and tries to touch him everywhere
8	MUSCLES	Her muscles relax, she is soft like silk and is completely relaxed or she bites and grabs his nipples
9	WHOLE BODY	She collapses, opens up, and completely surrenders in a total climax of rejuvenating emptiness

FEMALE EJACULATION

The fact that many women can ejaculate is news to many people but it is not a recent discovery. Aristotle referred to female ejaculation and ancient Taoists and Tantric adepts were also aware of its existence. Some women ejaculate every time they have intercourse and for others it only happens sometimes. And many women never ejaculate at all and still manage to have a good time.

The Taoists refer to fluids produced during sexual activity as the "three waters." The first water is the lubrication experienced during arousal; the second water consists of fluids emitted during orgasm; and the third is the female ejaculate released from the urethral sponge and is directly related to the stimulation of the G-spot (see page 52). However, for some women, G-spot stimulation is not necessary for orgasm with ejaculation. Some women have learned that bearing down at the point of orgasm leads to ejaculation. It is also thought that the stronger the PC muscle (see page 54), the more likely the possibility of ejaculation.

The fluid released during ejaculation has a watery texture and is clear or milky, depending on your diet and also where you are in your monthly cycle. The amount of fluid produced varies greatly from unnoticeable to a teaspoon to copious gushes or spurts. Some women, who have the ability to ejaculate copious amounts of fluid, often experience a sense of shame and embarrassment. It's certainly nothing to be embarrassed about. It's something to be celebrated!

Ejaculation may occur with stimulation of the inside of the vagina and the G-spot, it may accompany orgasm, or it may occur simply as a sign of intense sexual pleasure without orgasm. Perhaps knowing that it is a possibility will encourage you and your lover to explore it and expand your sexual repertoires. This will enhance your sexual response and allow you to let go, safe in the knowledge that you are not urinating.

Even if you do not have the ability to ejaculate, your capacity for giving and receiving pleasure will be more rewarding and your sexual pleasure will be enhanced by practicing your PC muscle exercises.

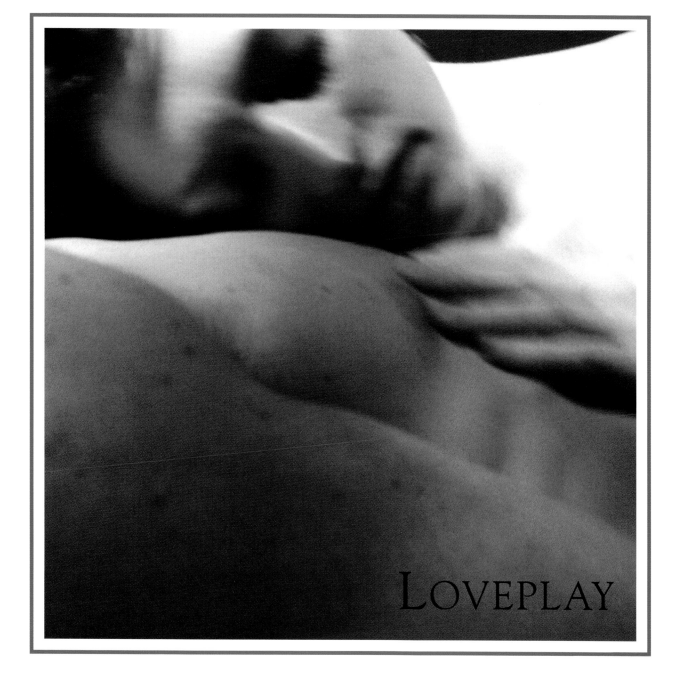

LOVEPLAY

THE VALUE OF LOVEPLAY

"...a sexual relationship without preliminaries is incomplete. Desire, affection, love create a lasting state of mind, through which the boy and girl, stimulated by caresses and kisses, abandon themselves wholeheartedly to the act of love."

RUPAGOSVAMI

In the West, we tend to view foreplay as the warm-up before intercourse, whereas in many Asian cultures it has traditionally been regarded as a complete and whole part of the sexual experience. I agree with the Asian view, and that is why I prefer to use the term "loveplay" rather than "foreplay." Foreplay implies activities that are only a lead-up to something else—either intercourse and/or orgasm—rather than activities that fully engage the participants in the here and now. When love is present and you are experiencing the continuum of moment-to-moment pleasure and surrendering to the moment, there is no future to look forward to or past to reflect upon.

It is really valuable during any act of love to remain completely and utterly in the present. One of the differences between making love and having sex is thought. If you are thinking, then you are not totally present and neither is love. Indulge in the actual physical sensations you experience in your body the moment that they happen. The greatest stimulation the body can receive is love.

Erotic possibilities outside intercourse include kissing and caressing, erotic massage, masturbation, and oral sex, as well as sexual games and toys. If you increase your sexual options, you will heighten your sexual response, enhance desire and passion, and deepen the intimacy between you and your lover.

Loveplay also introduces change and variety into lovemaking and prevents sex from becoming a routine, which can be a destructive factor in a relationship. It encourages lovers to discuss and experiment and to lose inhibitions, and presents them with ideas they may not have thought of

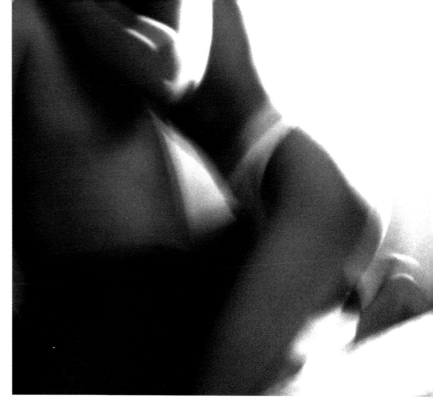

before. By engaging in more lengthy erotic give-and-take, without the goal of orgasm, levels of sexual excitement can expand, grow, and widen.

When you are able to appreciate sex and loving as an act of worship, you will know that kissing, touching, and caressing are all essential to the worship ritual. By touching and caressing each other you stay in touch with yourself and your lover. Through the caress, energy flows in and through our bodies, and keeps us alive, awake, appreciative, and grateful.

Caressing can be a gentle touching with the hands and fingers, perhaps accompanied by oils or creams. It can also consist of stroking, kissing, nuzzling, and licking with the lips and tongue. Or it can be accomplished through using the breath or a part of the anatomy—breasts or lingam, even toes or feet—to stroke your lover's body. It could even consist of rubbing entire bodies together, and it can be just as intimate when fully clothed as by meeting flesh with flesh.

SUCCESSFUL LOVEPLAY

It does not necessarily follow that sexual expertise ensures good lovemaking, and a sexual technician is not necessarily a good lover. Essential components of good lovemaking include compatibility between lovers and a similar and shared degree of commitment—whether for a night or for a lifetime. Another component is confidence in yourself, which ultimately produces confidence in your lover and sensitivity to his or her moods and reactions. However the most potent component of all is love.

Successful loveplay really has to be experienced as a time of mutual erotic pleasure or supreme worship, not a chore that must be performed in order to get to intercourse. And the sense of gently controlling and relishing your lover's enjoyment will extend and intensify your own pleasure. Of course,

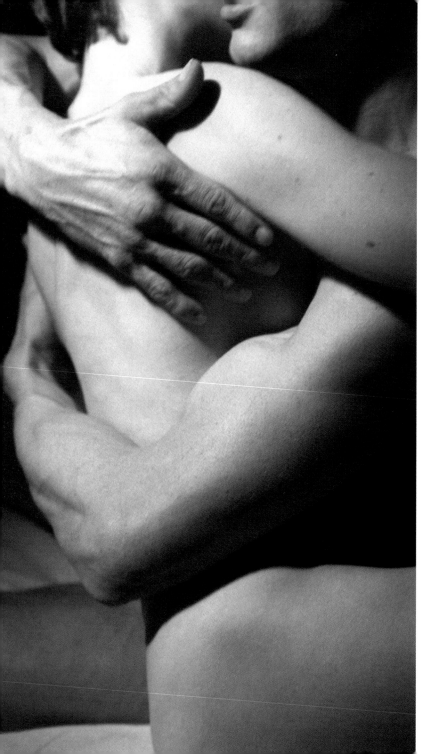

there will be times when a couple are both so aroused when they begin to make love that the woman wants her lover to enter her immediately. Sometimes nothing can be more exciting than this "can't wait" lovemaking, but arousal is usually a much slower process, particularly for a woman.

The rule for pleasing is very simple— don't force your lover to do anything that he or she finds distasteful or uncomfortable. Don't be afraid to ask for what you want or to ask your lover what he or she wants. Nobody is expected to have complete insight into someone else's desires, so communicate with one another and tell each other what gives you pleasure and what you find uncomfortable.

Man and woman are, in many ways, mysteries to one another, but how each obtains optimum sexual joy need not be a secret. You can unlock this mystery with communication, practice, and love, which are the keys to lasting sexual happiness with your partner.

BEAR IN MIND...

The erogenous zones (see pages 68 and 70) that play a crucial part in good loveplay are highly individual. What your ex-lover enjoyed may be very different to what your present lover loves. Explore your lover's body—every nook and cranny—to find out what turns him or her on. It is well worth the time and effort if it means a more exciting and erotic experience for both of you. Also, the value of personal cleanliness cannot be stressed enough. The anus, for example, is an extremely erotic area of the body—but only when it is completely clean and hygienic. You want to be able to explore, kiss, lick, squeeze, rub, and probe every part of each other's body without the slightest concern over hygiene, otherwise your lovemaking will be inhibited even before it starts.

The use of words, and sounds, during loveplay and lovemaking can contribute greatly to your lover's arousal. Talking also can bring an element of fun into loveplay, and if you can remain sensitive to each other's needs, you can interpret your lover's reactions, helping to dispel inhibitions and creating a mood of relaxation.

Biting has its place in loveplay, as does nipping, slapping, and scratching. Depending on your mood and what you like, a degree of pain can be exciting but is usually best confined to the less-sensitive areas of the body.

Next, I will discuss the erogenous zones, those parts of the body that respond particularly well to a lover's attention, and tell you what attention to apply. As a prelude, you can dwell on the following: The biggest erogenous zone of the body is the mind, and there's nothing more stimulating than anticipation.

LOVEPLAY TIPS
- Take your time.
- Relax into it.
- Savor every moment.
- Try a relaxed, leisurely massage for a gentle turn-on.
- Touching hair and skin creates an intimate atmosphere.
- Whole-body hugs generate warmth and a sense of reassurance.
- Lingering kisses and gentle nibbling of the earlobes are sure to arouse.
- Both sexes enjoy having their nipples gently caressed, licked, and sucked.
- A man will experience intense pleasure if you squeeze and stroke his lingam while he watches.
- A woman will enjoy having her pubic area stroked and her clitoris stimulated before any deeper exploration begins.

A MAN'S EROGENOUS ZONES

While it seems as if a man has only one erogenous zone—his genitals—it is probably just because nobody has ever bothered searching for more. Take the time to explore his body and you will most likely discover several areas that really turn him on.

Men are generally more susceptible to visual stimulation than women, an important point to bear in mind during loveplay. Generally, a man likes to be able to watch his lover and see what she is doing to him. If you sit astride your lover, facing him while touching and caressing him, then he can see you and what arouses you.

HEAD AND FACE
Unless he has an obsession about his hair always being perfectly in place, your lover will probably enjoy having his head massaged and fingers run through his hair. There's a biological reason for this—endorphins, the so-called pleasure hormones, are released in the brain when the scalp is massaged.

Kiss, lick, suck on, and nibble his earlobes. Make it subtle. You might try whispering or blowing or just breathing into his ear canal. The warm air can be very arousing. And when you are not gazing lovingly into your lover's eyes, gently brush his eyelids with your fingertips or tongue. Nibble or bite his nose gently and rub noses together, and don't just kiss his lips, devour them sensuously! Lick them, suck on them, kiss them soft, kiss them hard. Use the tip of your tongue on the roof of his mouth. Apparently, the lower lip of the male is linked to his lingam by an energy channel. Experiment!

HIS NECK
Kiss and lick the area under his jawbone and around his Adam's Apple. Alternate back and forth between his neck and his lips. Take long, deep sniffs or breathe on the back of his neck.

HIS FRONT
Just like women, men have sensitive nipples and many men get extremely aroused when their nipples are stroked, tweaked, flicked, pinched, licked, and even gently bitten. Stroking a man's belly and circling around his navel with the flat of your palm is another good way to arouse him.

BACK AND BOTTOM

Women tend to love men's muscular backs, and they also tend to ignore them during loveplay and lovemaking. Knead his back and shoulder muscles with your hands and kiss and lick up and down his spine. Rub his tailbone gently until it feels warm.

A man's buttocks and anal region have a lot of sensitive nerve endings. Caress and grab his bottom, then slide one finger between his buttocks and massage his anus.

HANDS AND FEET

Rotate and circle your middle finger around the center and mound of first one palm and then the other. Start off gently then massage more vigorously, and end by gently biting and sucking his thumbs and fingertips.

Many people find the whole idea of someone sucking on their toes or licking the bottom of their feet disgusting. But some men adore the special attention of a foot massage and get excited when a woman sucks, licks, and kisses their toes.

HIS GENITALS

Stroking the base of his lingam just above the scrotum can be quite arousing. The scrotum itself is extremely sensitive but you can caress and even lightly squeeze if he's not too delicate.

As for the lingam itself, the entire shaft loves to be stroked but it's the tip that has the most nerve endings. For best effect, it should be rubbed, gently flicked, sucked, and licked.

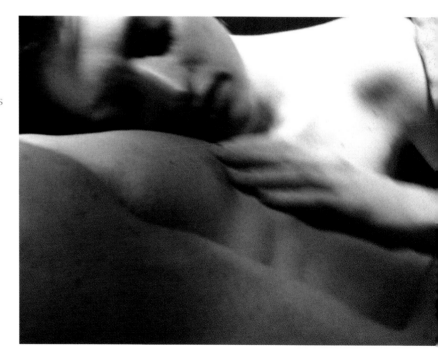

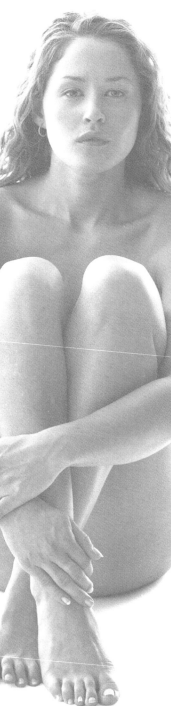

A WOMAN'S EROGENOUS ZONES

The main erogenous zones of a woman are similar to those of a man. Like those of a man, her most arousing spots are usually her nipples and genitals. But most of her other erogenous zones, such as her ears, neck, shoulders, hands, and feet are more sensitive than a man's are.

HEAD AND FACE

Because the highly pleasurable endorphins are released in a woman's brain when her scalp is massaged, I suggest either shampooing your lover's hair while she's bathing or showering, or offering to brush her hair. Not only will you be concentrating on one of her erogenous zones, but the special, seemingly nonsexual attention will probably make her melt.

Many women enjoy having their ears licked or kissed. Light stroking and nibbling of her earlobe and the outline of her ear are both pleasurable. Your lover will also like it when you whisper softly in her ears.

If you know how to touch her lips by kissing, licking, sucking, and gently biting, it is very possible that a kiss will open her up to more intensity. Use your lips, your tongue, and your teeth to play with her top and bottom lips, and then kiss her with absolute passion.

HER NECK

Just breathing on the nape of a woman's neck can be very arousing for her, as will using your tongue and teeth on it. Use your hands too; lift her hair up gently as you bring your mouth closer to her neck. Then gently pull on her hair to indicate your passion and desire for her.

BREASTS AND NIPPLES

Cupping her breasts, caressing them, gently fondling and squeezing them, pressing them together, and, of course, kissing, licking, and sucking them are all highly erotic for her. She will also enjoy it if you trace your fingertips around the outline of her breasts and around her nipples. The valley between her breasts is also a sensitive area, so give it some attention with your mouth, tongue, and fingers. Take care when you are handling your lover's breasts, especially before and during menstruation, because as well as being sexually sensitive they are easily hurt or bruised.

Her nipples, of course, also respond to touch. Squeeze or roll each nipple between thumb and forefinger, suck and roll your tongue around it, or flick the tip of it repeatedly with your tongue. Do remember to be gentle, because, like her breasts, her nipples can be easily hurt.

ARMS AND WRISTS

A woman's arms and wrists can be erotically sensitive to touch if it is light and gentle. Very lightly stroke the undersides of her forearms and wrists with your fingertips, or gently run your fingernails along them.

To include her underarm in your sensual stroking, extend her arm out and lightly slide your fingertips down the inside of it. Run your fingertips from her wrist up to her armpit, just barely touching her breast as you pass. She will also enjoy it if you nuzzle, lick, and nibble her wrists.

BELLY AND NAVEL

Many women love to have their bellies and navels tickled and caressed. Use your fingertips to lightly comb her abdomen in a back-and-forth motion. Then take one of your fingers and slowly and gently draw circles on her tummy and around her navel.

Next, place your hands on her waist, just below her ribs, and gently but firmly move your hands down over her belly toward her genitals—but stop before you get there. Instead of moving on to stimulate her genitals, which she might have been expecting, surprise her by using your lips and tongue to kiss and lick her navel. Vary the sensations by varying the speed and pressure of your kisses and licks.

INNER THIGHS AND KNEES

The insides of her thighs have many nerve endings, so this is an area highly sensitive to stroking, touching, and licking. Use your hands and tongue to massage and lightly caress them.

The thin, soft, sensitive skin behind the knees loves to be gently stroked and teased with fingernails. Because the nerves are so close to the surface here it is a very sensitive area. Your lover will find it surprisingly erotic and arousing when you gently lick or nibble on the backs of her knees.

"A man should gather from the actions of a woman of what disposition she is, and in what way she likes to be enjoyed."

KAMA SUTRA

BACK AND BOTTOM

Massage and caress her back muscles, using your fingernails and fingertips to lightly rake or comb up and down her spine and to rub her lower back. This can be done with her either lying down or sitting up with her back to you, or while she is straddled on top of you during intercourse. When it comes to soft, wet caresses, a woman's back is very sensitive, so make your way behind her and use your mouth to breathe heavily down the small of her back.

The many sensitive nerve endings in the buttocks make this a prime area to knead, squeeze, caress, lick, bite, and even to gently spank. Some women like having their buttocks licked, sucked, and penetrated with fingers, penis, or both.

Her Feet and Ankles

Many women enjoy having their feet and ankles touched, massaged, caressed, and nibbled, and even licked and sucked. Some women especially enjoy it when their lovers spend time caressing their soles, toes, and ankles. Because these zones can all be ticklish, the sensation of ticklishness can be pleasant for the recipient.

A foot massage can be an extremely relaxing and sensual experience for her, particularly if you learn to manipulate the reflexology pressure points. Also, try licking the bottoms of her feet and sucking on her toes, and lubricating your fingers with massage oil and sliding them between her toes.

Yoni and Clitoris

A woman's vulva, or the lips on the outside of her vagina, can be rubbed, kissed, licked, or lightly caressed. The clitoris is the most sensitive spot to focus on, and you can stimulate it by using your tongue or fingers or both simultaneously. Some women like to show their lovers the specific amount of pressure they enjoy.

The famous G-spot can be elusive and hard to find, however it is usually worth the effort. Locate it by placing a fingertip inside her vagina about two inches up. Then press the fingertip against the front wall of her vagina. She'll let you know when you find the spot (see also page 52). There are other areas inside women's vaginas that produce intense sexual feelings when stimulated. Once located, very gentle stimulation of them gives an incredibly pleasant, very unusual sensation and, if you hit the fabled G-spot, possibly even ejaculation.

Although it's usually quite evident whether or not she's enjoying it, be sensitive to how your lover moves and the patterns of her breathing, or simply ask her.

Making Love to a Woman

When you make love to a woman, whether you have intercourse or not, make good use of her erogenous zones to bring her to the highest levels of sexual arousal. Start off by kissing her with love and passion—sometimes a kiss can be orgasmic. Use your tongue to slowly arouse her senses. Look her in the eyes and slowly lick her lips with your wet tongue. Hold her face with your hands and kiss your way down from her lips to her chin. Then gently lift her face and begin sensually kissing, licking, and sucking on her neck.

Now head for other parts that you would typically leave out when it comes to sexual intercourse. Lick between her breasts while you firmly fondle and squeeze them, but don't start licking them as soon as you get there. Take your time to bring each other to the heights of sensual ecstasy.

Make your way down to her navel and slowly lick around it. Then gradually move over to her hips, where you can spend time slowly biting, nuzzling, and sucking on them.

Another very sensitive area of a woman's body is the inside of her thighs. Lick them lovingly, then open her legs wide and lick between her outer labia and her thighs.

Next, place your hands palms-up under her buttocks, and let her rest her feet on your shoulders while her legs are in a butterfly (spread-eagle) position. Use the tip of your tongue to lightly tap her clitoris, then start kissing it slowly, like you would her mouth.

By this time, if you have remained sensitive, her heightened state of arousal will have turned the whole of her body into one big erogenous zone.

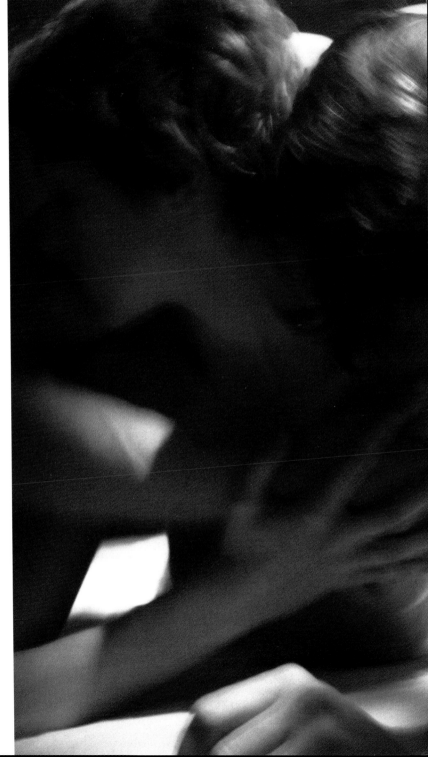

INTIMATE TOUCH

> *"From among the senses, the sense of touch pervades all the others and has the mind inherent in it."*
>
> CHARAKA SAMHITA

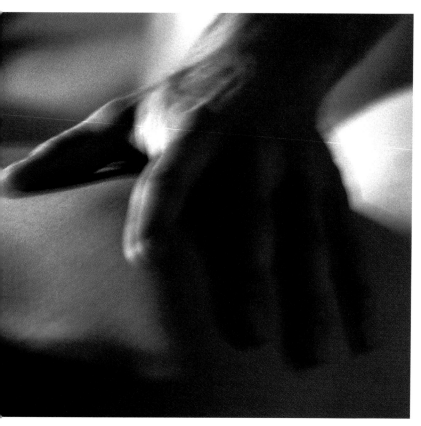

Touch is the only way we physically connect with one another and we never grow out of our need for it; touch is as essential as food or water. Touch can be healing, nurturing, and exciting, and can communicate feelings and emotions on a deep and immediate level. A gentle stroking touch can change your whole state of being almost immediately—and for the better. Anger, tenderness, love, tension, support, care, desire—all come across with the slightest physical contact. Loving touch can rejuvenate, make you feel good and worthwhile, lower stress and improve your immune system.

Sexual touch is the most intimate way of touching. With it you explore your lover's skin, experiencing and feeling the softness and hardness of the different patterns and textures of the body. Touch also helps to establish trust and becomes a mutual voyage of discovery. To have permission to touch someone intimately and sexually is a special gift and a privilege.

Using Massage

Massage (including erotic massage—see page 78) is not only a simple way of relaxing the body it is also one of the most direct methods of establishing deep communication with one another. It can express love and compassion, and demonstrates our sensitivity and awareness. Using it, you can discover the pleasure of giving without demands or expectations. In honoring your lover with your touch, both of you will gain balance in mind, body, and spirit.

Like lovemaking, all massage needs to be reciprocal—not necessarily at the same time—just in terms of taking turns to give and receive. Healing and relaxing massage is an extremely valuable and pleasurable tool to share with your lover and it can become an integral part of your relationship. As a means of loveplay, it helps to clear the body of accumulated tensions, attunes your bodies to one another, and brings them to the state of relaxation that is essential for lovemaking.

The secret of the effectiveness of massage lies in the intention with which it is given. It calls for concentration and confidence from the person performing the massage, and trust and surrender from the person being massaged.

Affectionate touch and sexual touch are different and it is important to know which you are giving or asking for. There is "giving touch" and there is "taking touch." Be clear about which you are doing and which your lover wants. The intention must be obvious before you begin, to allow the massage to remove energy blockages or obstacles in your lover and invigorate and charge his or her body with positive energy.

Make massage a ritual on the full or new moon, an equinox, or solstice. Offer a massage as a gift to your beloved, for a birthday or anniversary. Set aside a specific day or evening or just be spontaneous.

Communication

Whether verbal or nonverbal, communication between giver and receiver is important and necessary, especially in the beginning. However, it is also vital that you do not criticize what your lover is doing. Find a loving and encouraging way to make requests or suggestions as to what feels good.

It is also important for the person receiving the massage to be comfortable about making requests and comments. He or she must always feel free to mention anything that is getting in the way of his or her comfort and pleasure. It ensures that the receiver is getting the kind of strokes and stimulation that he or she likes. In turn, this motivates the giver and ensures that he or she is not giving anything unwanted.

Many sexual difficulties stem from one or other of the partners worrying—maybe that a lover is getting tired of pleasuring, or that the pleasuring is not being enjoyed. Letting your receiving partner know verbally and nonverbally that you're actively enjoying giving pleasure can be a powerful aphrodisiac.

As the receiver, the more you are able to surrender, the more beneficial and intimate the experience will be. Sexy compliments and eye contact will encourage your lover. Any requests you may make, such as to go to the bathroom, for touch to be harder or lighter, to take a break or stop, or for the heat to be turned up, will be signs that levels of communication and trust are high. They are also signs that you are paying attention to your feelings, which is the secret to experiencing greater pleasure.

Other than expressing what you like and what you want, and how you want to receive it, focus on using your breath and sounds as well as words. Make noises of pleasure so your lover knows that you are appreciating and enjoying being touched.

Making sounds also increases the pleasure you feel, and helps you to remain present in the sensations. It stops your mind from wandering off and being distracted by thoughts, and so wasting the experience.

RELEASING EMOTIONS

Some people find that sex and/or pleasure can bring up difficult emotional issues. Our bodies hold memories, both painful and joyous ones. The painful ones can create blockages, which can stop the flow of energy as well as inhibit the release of an orgasm.

If your lover starts crying, or appears to be in a distressed state while being touched, it is usually best to just be there for that person. Reassure your lover that he or she is safe, and that it is all right to cry (possibly while you hold him or her) rather than trying to discuss what is going on or engage in rational problem-solving. Asking your lover what he or she needs rather than assuming too much is also a good idea.

CONSCIOUS BREATHING

Regular, conscious breathing is a powerful way to enhance both relaxation and erotic massage. If the receiving lover forgets to breathe regularly, the massaging lover can remind him or her by breathing rhythmically and audibly. Some lovers find that synchronizing the breathing between the two of them leads to wonderful and intimate sensations.

Deep exhalation is as important as inhalation and is a form of surrender. The stronger the exhalation, the more the lover is able to surrender during lovemaking, and is able to give and receive love with profound feeling. When you combine massage with controlled breathing it becomes more and more blissful for both of you.

LUBRICATION

Make sure your massage oils are warm before using them. You can warm them by putting the bottles in a basin of warm water or running hot water over them for a few minutes. For a sensual body massage, try using cornstarch rather than massage oil to ensure a feather-light touch. Cornstarch feels like cool raindrops when it is sprinkled on and makes the skin feel incredibly silky.

For genital massage on a man, use a light, nonsticky oil such as sesame, sunflower, grape seed, safflower, or pure coconut. For a woman, use a water-based lubricant when giving a genital massage to avoid encouraging vaginal infections. Always insure that the water-based lubricant you choose does *not* contain Nonoxynol-9, which can cause irritation.

COCOONING

When you have finished the massage it is nice to fold a sheet and/or blanket covering over your lover and allow him or her to remain with a quiet, still, warm, and safe feeling.

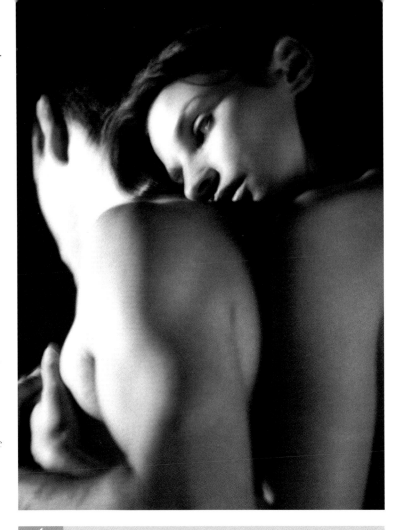

"Relax and feel everyone so openly that you feel as everyone, as their shape, as their fear, as their deep heart's love. As everyone, open and breathe. As the shape of the entire moment, open and breathe. If closure remains, feel, breathe, and open again, without end."

DAVID DEIDA

EROTIC MASSAGE

"No matter what you are feeling on the surface, deep down you want to give and receive unbounded love."

DAVID DEIDA

Erotic massage creates eroticism and sexual arousal by the combined use of massage strokes and stimulation of the erogenous zones. During the process of giving an erotic massage, either you, your lover, or both of you might become aroused, or fall asleep, or burst out in laughter, giggles, or tears. And you might or might not make love before, during, or after it, or reach orgasm, or ejaculate.

Erotic massage is, of course, a wonderful prelude to intercourse. However, it's a good idea to let go of the notion that when you start touching each other it has to end in intercourse. In having intercourse, you may miss out on many other pleasures.

What is important is that you allow each feeling, each moment, to unfold itself fully and at its own speed, while you remain totally in the sensational present. Stay completely in the moment, utterly immersed in the wonderful sensations of what you are giving or receiving.

TIPS FOR SUCCESS
- Try to keep in constant contact with your partner's body while you are giving the massage. Maintain a continuous flow, blending your movements smoothly together.
- Vary the pressure, tempo, and rhythm; ask the recipient if he or she wants it harder or softer, deeper or lighter.
- Breathe long, slow, deep breaths and remind the recipient to breathe too.
- No amount of technique makes up for a lack of soul. Put your heart into it.

WHAT YOU WILL NEED
- A willing recipient.
- Clean hands, clean trimmed nails, and clean bodies. Bath or shower together.
- A beautiful, clean, and warm space, free from drafts and, if outside, free of insects and out of strong sunlight.
- A natural massage oil (not mineral-based), or a water-based lubricant.
- Towels, a sheet, and/or blankets to lie on and be cocooned in.
- Soft pillows and cushions for comfort and support.
- Gentle music, incense, flowers, and soft lighting or candles.
- A vibrator, feathers, and a silk scarf to use as a blindfold.
- Items that stimulate the senses (bells, rattles, essential oils).

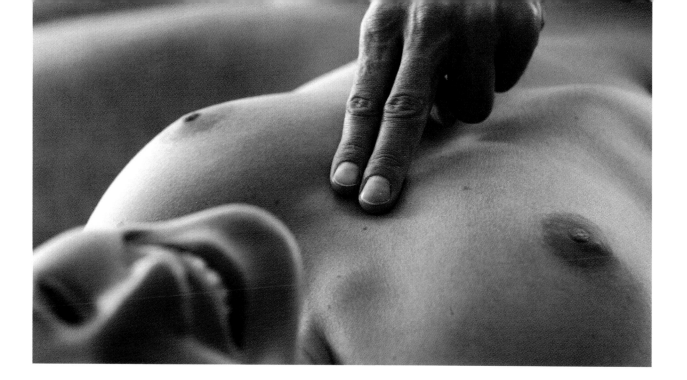

MAKING MASSAGE A RITUAL

To make your erotic massage really special, turn it into an energizing ritual. To begin the ritual, use the first two fingers of your left hand to touch your lover's head, forehead, eyes, throat, earlobes, breasts, upper arms, heart, navel, thighs, genitals, and feet. The touching will charge these places with the vital energy of transformation.

Rub your hands together to warm them, then lay them on your lover's head or on his or her feet. Harmonize your breathing with your lover's, and use breath control to help with concentration. Inhale deeply, hold the breath without tensing your body for a moment or two, and then fully exhale. The key to creative massage is to channel energy from your whole body, out through your hands. Consciously draw the energy up through your body and visualize it being emitted through your fingertips. Bear in mind that touch has a great potential for both healing and vitalization.

CREATIVE MOUTH MASSAGE

With your tongue, explore, lick, and kiss every part of your lover's body—the skin between the fingers, the crook of the elbows, the armpits, the backs of the knees, and the soles of clean feet. Suck on the fingers and toes. Use your

Begin your massage ritual by using the first two fingers of your left hand to energize your lover's body.

fingers as well as your lips and tongue to explore your lover's mouth. Look into your lover's eyes or keep your eyes closed to emphasize, sharpen, and hone your sense of touch. Explore the whole body before you include the genitals.

Experiment with different mouth temperatures while kissing, licking, and sucking each other. Alternate between having ice cubes and a hot liquid in your mouth to create exciting and surprising sensations. Another effective technique is to place a single drop of peppermint oil on your tongue. Lick it onto your lover's lingam or yoni to create an arousingly tingling sensation.

FULL-BODY MASSAGE

Developed in the harems of the East, the full-body or Oriental massage is having the whole body massaged with the body of another. It involves the receiver being rubbed all over by the giver. Both bodies are lubricated with oil or lather. The giver lies on top and uses different parts of his or her body to massage, stimulate, and invigorate the body of the other. The elbows, knees, thighs, breasts, chin, forehead, feet, and other body parts are all used.

This kind of massage is extremely sensuous for both partners, and it can be a wonderful prelude to lovemaking or done simply as an act of loving service in itself.

GENITAL MASSAGE

Our genitals are very potent generators of energy. When the lingam and yoni are stimulated, the energy spreads throughout the rest of the body. You do not need to rely solely on technique; be intuitive and spontaneous and feel confident, even though you may not be! Remember to stimulate the entire lingam or entire yoni to produce healing effects on the whole body.

The following are some of the most effective and popular strokes for lingam and yoni massage. Experiment with some or all of them, and use at least two or three different strokes during each massage.

LINGAM MASSAGE

When you massage your lover's lingam, he does not need an erection for it to feel good. Some of the strokes actually feel better when the lingam is soft.

The basic principle of lingam massage is to slow down, stop, or change what you are doing just before ejaculation becomes inevitable. The best way to accomplish this is for the man to give a signal just before this point is reached.

Although delaying ejaculation is desirable for maximizing pleasure, many lovers do like to finish the massage with an ejaculation because it provides a considerable spark of pleasure. However it can leave men too fatigued to enjoy the rest of the experience, or without enough energy left for massaging their lover. Opposite-sex partners who like to finish male genital massage with ejaculation may choose to offer the woman her massage first.

There are many different massage strokes that feel good on male genitals. Unless he indicates otherwise, it's usually safe to assume that firm and consistent stroking will feel best. With your lover lying naked on his back and you comfortably positioned beside him, begin by resting your left hand on his head, with the palm on his forehead and the fingers on the top of his head. Rest your right hand on his pelvic area with the palm covering his scrotum.

GENITAL REFLEXOLOGY

If you are familiar with foot reflexology, you will know that the soles of the feet contain the endings of nerves and meridians and that various points on the feet correlate with various parts of the body. You will also know that by massaging these points, you can bring energy and healing to their related organs.

The Taoists discovered that each part of the genitals, male and female, corresponds with another part of the body, and that the reflexology points are stronger on the sex organs than on the feet or hands.

Through manual stimulation, oral sex, and intercourse, you can directly stimulate a organ that needs strengthening or is in need of healing. You can also stimulate and revitalize the entire body with the possibility of experiencing a more intense whole-body orgasm.

During intercourse, when the lingam penetrates all the way into the yoni, the reflexology points of the lingam unite with the reflexology points in the yoni. In this way, heart is aligned with heart, lungs with lungs, and so on. Two lovers stimulating each other in this way has to be the most pleasurable form of reflexology! This is how two bodies become one.

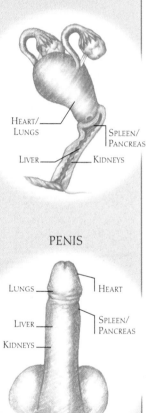

VAGINA

HEART/ LUNGS

SPLEEN/ PANCREAS

LIVER

KIDNEYS

PENIS

LUNGS

HEART

LIVER

SPLEEN/ PANCREAS

KIDNEYS

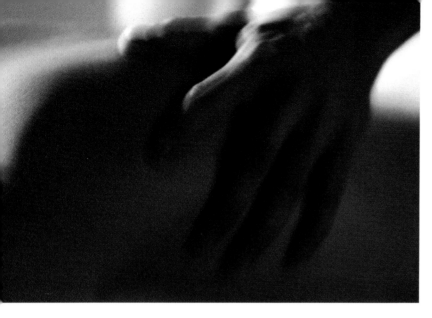

lingam. Put your other hand around the neck of the lingam (just below the head), and use your fingertips as if squeezing half an orange on a juicer while you slide the other hand up and down. Vary the pressure and the speed and ask your lover what he prefers.

THE FRENULUM STROKE

The underside of the head of the lingam is called the frenulum and is one of the most sensitive parts of a man's genitals. Rub your thumbs one at a time along the underside of the head of his lingam over the frenulum.

THE CLOCKWORK STROKE

Gently use one hand to stretch the foreskin down along the shaft of the lingam and hold it at its base. Using your thumb and index finger of your other hand, form a circle just below the head of the lingam and rotate in a clockwise direction as far as your wrist will turn. Repeat several times.

THE DESCENDING STROKE

Using plenty of oil and alternating hands, make ten downward strokes on the lingam and ten upward strokes. Practice stroking using different rhythms and check the pressure with your lover. Then follow ten strokes by nine strokes upward and nine strokes downward all the way to one up and one down.

ANOINTING STROKE

With the fingers of your left hand tight together, pour a little oil over the back of that hand. Quickly place your right hand, with your fingers slightly spread, onto the scrotum and underside of the lingam. Open the fingers of your left hand so that the oil seeps through the fingers. Alternating your hands, spread the oil with a pulling motion.

Starting at the perineum, slide your hands up over the scrotum and along the sensitive underside of the lingam. Keep the strokes long and smooth, with greater pressure on the perineum than on the scrotum and lingam.

THE JUICING STROKE

Hold the lingam at its base with one hand. If your lover has a foreskin, gently ease it down to expose the head of his

THE SCROTUM STROKE

Using your thumb, index, and middle fingers, encircle the scrotum (be careful not to squeeze the testicles). Now move the scrotum up and down as your other hand strokes up and down on the shaft of the lingam. Vary the amount of pressure against the base of the lingam.

THE HEALING STROKE

Bring one hand down, stroking the lingam from the tip of the head all the way to the base. When it hits the base, release it. Meanwhile bring your other hand to the top of the lingam and repeat the stroke, creating a constant stroking motion.

THE SURPRISE STROKE

Take the lingam in one hand and gently, sensuously caress it for about ten seconds, then give it one quick up-and-down stroke. Repeat the sensuous caressing for about ten seconds using slow up-and-down strokes, and then give the lingam two quick up-and-down strokes. Repeat the caressing, then give three quick strokes, and so on.

THE SPREADING STROKE

With the lingam resting on the belly, cup the scrotum with one hand. Glide the heel of the palm of your other hand up and down the underside of the lingam all the way to the tip.

ROLLING AND TICKLING STROKE

With your lover lying on his back, legs apart, kneel between his legs. Hold his scrotum between your fingers and thumbs and roll the testicles gently, slowly, and lightly with the pads of your fingertips. After a few minutes, put your hands underneath his testicles and with light pressure for more exquisite sensation, tickle them with the pads of your fingertips.

THE SPIRAL STROKE

This is a good technique if your lover is soft or has difficulty getting an erection. Hold the base of his lingam with one hand and take a firm hold of it with the other. Starting at the base, slide your hand to the tip along the length of the shaft, using a spiral stroke like a corkscrew motion. When you reach the glans, use the palm of your hand to caress the entire surface.

THE FIRE STROKE

Imagine you have a stick between your hands and are trying to start a fire by rolling it with your palms. With fingers straight and hands well-lubricated, hold the palms against each side of his lingam. Using a rolling, rubbing motion, start at the base of his lingam and slide up and down, keeping the rhythm and motion consistent. Start slowly and gradually build pressure and speed.

Yoni Massage

Offer your lover a yoni massage as a sensual gift without the pressure to make love at the end. The focus of this type of massage is not on having an orgasm, but she should feel free to have all the orgasms she wishes. As women can sometimes enjoy stimulation all the way through one orgasm and into the next, there is little or no need for them to hold back in any way. Having orgasms in a series can cause arousal levels to stay very high for a long time.

But before you begin her yoni massage, pay some attention to the rest of her body. Ask her to lie face-down, then massage the back of her body using stretches, vibrations, glides, circles, and kneading. Brush her skin with your fingertips, massage her scalp, and pinch her fingertips and toes. Then repeat this massage on her front.

Ways to Stimulate Her

Women often vary considerably in what type of sexual stimulation they like, and how they like it done. Female arousal usually takes longer to build, and can often last longer and be more intense than that which men commonly experience. Please be aware that clitoral stimulation and vaginal penetration usually feel much more exciting when a woman is already in a fairly high state of arousal and well lubricated.

- It is best to begin with gentle stroking, then ask her to tell you which strokes she prefers and to guide your hand to which pressure she prefers.
- A common preference is to begin the massage with gentle rubbing over the entire yoni, then to follow this with clitoral stimulation. Finish off with G-spot stimulation or G-spot and clitoral stimulation.
- Keep a regular rhythm going, rather than stopping and starting and chopping and changing too much.
- To add to her pleasure while massaging her yoni, glide your other hand over the rest of her body, caressing her breasts, teasing her nipples, massaging her perineum, and stroking her face.
- Experiment with some or all of the strokes, adapting them where necessary to suit her preferences.
- Use plenty of lubrication—it is better to have too much than not enough.
- For most of the strokes, she should lie naked on her back with her legs flat or slightly bent, and let her legs fall open naturally to the side. You should kneel comfortably, positioned between her thighs or beside her.
- Begin by resting your left hand on her head, with the palm on her forehead and the fingers on the top of her head. Rest your right hand on her pelvic area with the palm on her yoni.

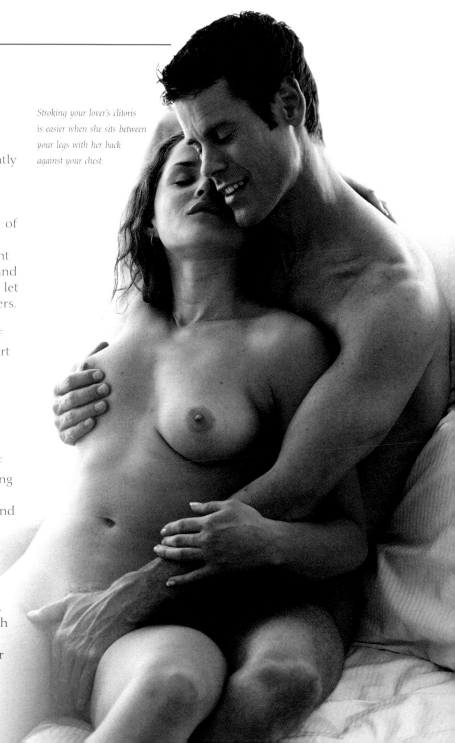

THE WAKE-UP STROKES

Gently tug on her pubic hair to stimulate her pubic region. Then part her lips and blow very softly and gently into her yoni.

ANOINTING STROKE

Pour warmed lubricant over the back of your left hand, keeping the fingers tightly closed. Quickly place your right hand palm-upward under her yoni, and open the fingers of your left hand to let the lubricant seep through your fingers. Alternating your hands, spread the lubricant with a pulling up motion of long, slow strokes from the lower part of the yoni, up over the clitoris and pubic bone, and back down again.

AS SHE LIKES IT

Ask her how she like her clitoris massaged, then do it. Be sure to incorporate massaging other areas of her body whenever possible, spreading the energy down her thighs and legs and up her body to her heart, face, and scalp, and the crown of her head.

THE CLITORAL STROKE

For this stroke, you might like to sit behind your lover with your back propped up or leaning against a wall. Your lover sits between your legs with her back against your chest. In this position, you can encircle her in your

Stroking your lover's clitoris is easier when she sits between your legs with her back against your chest.

arms and touch her breasts as you caress her yoni, and kiss her neck. Focus your stroking on and around the clitoris, which is just beneath where the inner lips merge together at the upper part of the vulva.

ROCK AROUND THE CLIT CLOCK

Gliding a lubricated finger softly and rhythmically around her clitoris will almost always make her feel good. With your index finger or using one or two fingers, slowly massage tiny circles around her clitoris, circling several times in each direction and stopping at every one of the twelve "hours."

THE LIP STROKES

Stroke her pubic hair and genital area with soft, gentle motions. Use the pads of your fingers to gently stroke and "tap" her outer lips, keeping a regular and consistent rhythm.

Sitting between her open thighs, gently massage the lips of her yoni with lubricated fingers, and delicately tug or stretch them away from her yoni. Pinch her lips between thumb and forefinger and then softly rub them together.

Use the knuckles of your index and middle fingers or your thumb and forefinger to gently knead her outer lips backward and forward. Massage downward from the top, where the clitoris meets the lips, and roll the lips between your knuckles with a firm and gentle pressure, toward her anus. Then with a thumb on one side and your index finger on the other side, very gently squeeze and slide off the edge of the lip. Alternate your hands and continue this series of strokes along the entire length of each lip.

ENTERING THE TEMPLE GATES

Some women find that clitoral orgasms feel better if their yonis are penetrated either with fingers or an appropriately-sized dildo—although penetration of any kind usually only feels good when the woman is in a state of arousal.

Ask her permission before you enter the temple gates of her yoni. Use lots of lubrication, and with one finger tickle the vaginal opening as lightly as possible. Make her hungry.

To enter the temple gates, keep one hand on her abdomen or heart and insert the forefinger of your other hand ever so slowly into her yoni. Hold still, with no movement. Just be there. Then slowly glide you finger in and out. Add your index finger if desired.

THE FOUR DIRECTIONS

Using two fingers, press firmly up, then to one side, then down, and finally to the other side. Repeat this pattern eight times clockwise then eight times counterclockwise.

Twist and Shout

Using one or more fingers, massage in and out of the vagina while twisting at the wrist.

G-spot Strokes

When you massage your lover's G-spot, pressing on the spot can be intensely arousing for her, but a gentle, beckoning, stroking motion is often far more pleasurable than pressing hard and constantly. In general, remember that it's the pads of your fingers that should be touching the spot during these massage stokes, and G-spot stimulation usually only feels good when the woman is aroused.

One easy way to stimulate the G-spot is with your lubricated index and middle fingers together. Begin with your index finger. Make rhythmic gestures inside her yoni with a "come hither" motion. Alternatively, rub the G-spot in a circular fashion. Another approach is to rotate your fingers inside her vagina, with even pressure on all areas of it.

The Double-action Stroke

While stimulating her G-spot, apply pressure and make circular motions in both directions. Simultaneously, use your thumb to make small circles on the clitoris or move your fingers directly backward and forward over it. Then alternate between G-spot stimulation and clitoral stimulation, 10 seconds for each. You can suggest that she contract and release her PC muscle at the same time—the feeling is fantastic!

Healing Thrusts

When your partner is highly aroused, she might enjoy good, hard, deep, vigorous in-and-out penetration with two or more fingers. Encourage her to stay relaxed, to let go, and to make audible sounds when she exhales.

The Vibrator Stroke

Vibrators generally work best externally, on or near the clitoris. If the vibration is too intense, switch to a lower speed or put a piece of silk or soft cloth between the vibrator and her clitoris. To begin with, she should guide your hand and the vibrator to show you the pressure she prefers. For added pleasure, use the vibrator on the clitoris while you penetrate her yoni with your fingers.

Leaving the Temple

At the end of the massage, stay present. With your hand inside her yoni, slow down to no movement. Just be there. Withdraw your fingers as slowly as possible. Wrap your lover in a warm towel or sheet and allow her to savor the afterglow for as long as she wishes.

THE KISS

"When a woman is excited with passion, she should cover her lover's eyes with her hands and, closing her own eyes, thrust her tongue into his mouth. She should move it to and fro and in and out, with a pleasant motion suggestive of more intimate forms of enjoyment to come."

ANANGA RANGA

When lovers kiss, their purpose is to draw close to each other, to develop love and mutual trust, and to arouse sensuousness and pleasure. Lips are one of the most sensitive areas of the body and play an important role in lovemaking. The kiss is the gateway to bliss and impassioned experience. It provokes erotic desire and excites the heart, yet in many long-term relationships kissing is quite often the first thing to be neglected or forgotten.

Kissing is an art—and an art to be cultivated. The face is the center of your senses—sight, sound, taste, touch, and smell. The mouth and lips are extremely sensitive, so when you are kissing, you are the closest you can be with anyone and completely in each other's space.

In the tongue and lips we have erotic organs with the characteristics of both the lingam and yoni yet without their limitations. The lips and tongue are controlled by voluntary muscles, which means we can kiss as much and for as long as we want to even when we are physically exhausted.

There are many different types of kiss and a deep, inspired, erotic kiss is a world away from a formal, tight-lipped, closed-mouth peck! Kissing can be more intimate than intercourse, and in India and China the sensual kiss is considered the epitome of eroticism and as such is practiced in absolute privacy.

Kissing requires much less energy than lovemaking and can be enjoyed whenever two people wish. It also is an extremely erotic prelude to lovemaking, and continues to arouse and express pleasure during and after sex. Whether you progress from kissing to lovemaking or not, kissing is a wonderful exchange of intimacy, love, and trust.

WAYS TO KISS

When kissing, keep your mouth and jaw relaxed and use your tongue to explore your lover's lips, mouth, teeth, and tongue. When you kiss, become the kiss, and for each kiss you receive, offer one in return.

Tantra teaches that the upper lip of a woman is linked to her clitoris by a subtle nerve channel. Similarly, the lower lip of a man is linked to his lingam. So when a man stimulates the upper lip of a woman by gentle nibbling and sucking on it, while she gently uses her teeth and tongue to play with his lower lip, they can create waves of pleasure that are very arousing for both of them.

Be aware of this the next time you kiss. Also be aware of your lover's scent, which is easy to detect when you are kissing. Each man and woman has a scent of his or her own, and there is a connection between body odor and sexual excitation. As your lover becomes more aroused, his or her body scent will change, and at the moment of orgasm man and woman give off a particular smell.

Such smells excite you and increase your erotic ability. And although the variations are subtle, if you learn to be sensitive to the slight changes of scent they will give you a clear indication of your lover's state of arousal.

> *"Between the lips and the bottom of the gums, there is a highly sensitive area, which in a certain way, is similar to the one between the lips and the interior of the yoni. At the tongue's contact, a powerful current of excitation appears in the lips and throat, strengthening sexual desire."*
>
> KAMA SUTRA

The sounds, however small, that are made by your lover while kissing are also significant. They will also give you an indication of your lover's arousal.

Passionate and sensual kissing does not need to be restricted to your lover's mouth. Use your lips and tongue to explore every part of his or her body—eyelids, ears, and neck are especially sensitive. Move your hands on your lover's body or caress his or her face while kissing. This will to add to the sensuousness of the experience, and touching your lover's lips with your fingertips or sucking your lover's finger while kissing can be deeply erotic.

You should think of everything you do with your lover as something you are receiving. So when kissing, try to experience it as what you are receiving and how you are receiving it—the feel of your lover's kiss, mouth, lips, and tongue; the softness, the texture—drinking in your lover's very essence.

KISSING SWEET

Good oral hygiene is essential to the enjoyment of the deep sexuality and intimacy of sensual kissing. Clean teeth and fresh breath make the whole experience infinitely more harmonious and appealing.

The value of scrupulous personal hygiene cannot be stressed enough. When you are with your lover you want to feel that there are no parts of the body "out of bounds" to receiving pleasure and love. The realization that you will not being able to explore your lover's body in its entirety for hygiene reasons inhibits lovemaking even before it starts. The ideal is to be able to use your mouth, lips, and tongue to kiss, lick, blow, caress, nibble, and suck all over your lover's body without the slightest concern.

THE *KAMA SUTRA* SUGGESTS DIFFERENT WAYS OF KISSING

NOMINAL
The man seizes the woman's head with his hands and applies his mouth forcefully on hers, but without violence.

VIBRANT
The man seeks to insert his lip into the woman's mouth, but does not attempt to seize her mouth. Since her lips tremble, however, she does not allow him to seize her lower lip.

RUBBING
Holding her lover loosely, the woman closes her eyes and covers his eyes with her hands. She then rubs her lover's lips with her tongue.

THE AWAKENING
When one of a couple returns home late and kisses the sleeping partner, his or her intention is clear. This kind of kiss is called the awakening kiss.

THE INFLAMER
In order to arouse desire, seeing the mouth of one's sleeping lover, a man or woman embraces his or her lover and wakes the lover with a kiss, so that she or he immediately understands the other's intentions.

THE ENCOURAGEMENT
When a lover seems distracted by music or reading, or is in a bad mood, or indifferent to his or her lover, or shows interest in other individuals, or stays offended after a quarrel, in order to attract the lover's attention, appease the quarrel, shake off the indifference, the partner must embrace his or her lover, which is known as the kiss of encouragement.

SPECIAL KISSES
Special kisses consist of embracing different parts of the body and are:

DEVOURING
The forehead, chin, armpits, and below the breasts are tickled and lightly kissed.

EQUAL
Both partners are seated or lying next to each other, and kiss or nibble each other's thighs, chest, armpits, and pubis, neither too hard nor too soft.

PRESSED
Breasts, cheeks, buttocks, and navel are seized, pressed, and kneaded.

DELICATE
The eyes, neck, breasts, buttocks, and back are lightly tickled.

ORAL LOVING

Generally, the one erotic art that both lovers want more of—oral loving—requires a higher level of skill than most other aspects of lovemaking. However, it is a skill well worth mastering. Tongues are usually softer, wetter, more agile, and warmer than hands, and genitals respond readily to heat. Oral loving involves more technique, more sensitivity, and more practice than intercourse. The good news is that you need no special talent to progress other than willingness and a desire for openness.

As in mouth-to-mouth kissing, keep your face, jaw, and mouth relaxed and make sure your mouth is not dry. Swirling your tongue around your mouth and pressing it against your soft palate will increase saliva flow.

Verbal communication is important; tell each other what gives you pleasure in terms of rhythm and pressure. Also be aware of nonverbal clues, for example when your lover shifts his or her body posture to increase stimulation to a particular area.

And remember cleanliness. Good hygiene is essential if you want oral loving to be enjoyable for both of you. Washing each other before you begin will ensure that you both have the confidence to explore one another fully.

YONI KISSING

In Eastern cultures and Tantric rituals, the yoni is considered the most sacred part of a woman's body, worthy of both honor and worship. The yoni represents the source of life and is the physical representation of woman's mystery. It is a holy shrine, and man is the worshiper at that shrine.

When a woman's lover experiences her shrine as a meditation, touches it, tastes it, smells it, and enters it, something magical happens. As he worships at the Gateway of Life—in full consciousness and awareness, with deep reverence and awe, in love transcending every thought and every feeling—then man and woman as separate beings vanish, and the mystical union occurs. It is a woman's pleasure to receive such love, a man's pleasure to give it.

For many people, fear of the odor and taste of a woman is the chief barrier to yoni kissing. Every woman has her own scent and it changes according to where she is in her monthly cycle. It can also be influenced by what she eats and drinks. If your lover is clean and in good health, her taste and smell should not be unpleasant. Suggesting a shared shower or bath before lovemaking is a tactful approach and can be a very erotic invitation.

Ways to Kiss

Yoni kissing can be performed in various positions. Some women like to lie on their backs, some like to sit at the edge of the bed with their lovers kneeling between their legs, and some like it standing. Another popular position is for the man to lie on his back and the woman to kneel above him, then lower herself down to his mouth. In this position, the man can support his neck with a pillow, so as to enjoy the pleasure of a view of his partner's breasts while she has the control over pressure and position.

Whatever position you choose to end up in, begin by kissing, fondling, and caressing her entire body with your hands, breath, mouth, lips, and tongue. Try kissing and licking her ankles and the soles of her feet, or sucking her toes. Then stimulate her breasts and kiss and lick your way slowly up the insides of her legs and the backs of her knees. Tease her by kissing and licking her inner thighs and try gently blowing some air over her yoni.

Familiarize yourself with the whole of her genital area. Tell her you find her yoni sexy and you really want to explore it. Use lots of saliva over the whole yoni area and use the whole surface of the flat of your tongue. Begin with indirect stimulation, by kissing, licking, and nuzzling her pubic area.

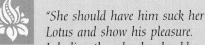

"She should have him suck her Lotus and show his pleasure. Inhaling the odor, he should enter with his tongue, searching for the Red and White secretions. Then she should say to him, 'Eat my essence! Drink the Waters of Release! O Son, be a slave as well as a father and lover!'"

CHANDAMAHAROSANA TANTRA

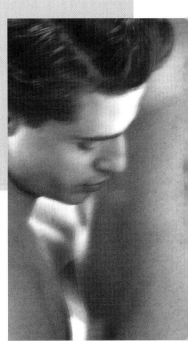

Then gently probe with your tongue and locate her yoni opening and her clitoris. Suck gently on her labia.

As she becomes more aroused, experiment with tensing your tongue and teasing her by running its tip around her clitoris and along either side of its shaft. A slurping action also works well. Then concentrate on the bud of her clitoris. Suck and massage it gently. Go in circles, up and down, or flick lightly back and forth. Gentle nibbling, sucking, and licking with the lips and tongue will make her feel good. Vary the speed and pressure of your actions and see how she responds. Ask her what she likes.

Next, gently slide the hood of her clitoris back to reveal more of this jewel. Make circles with your tongue around the edge of the clitoris and stroke up and down with it. Rhythmic stimulation combined with a gradual build-up is what feels best. Always be sensitive to her body language and her responses, and let her know how much you too are enjoying it. That reassurance will help her to relax and enjoy it even more.

You can also use your tongue to penetrate her—just make it rigid and plunge it in. Move it in and out or keep it still and move your head, stimulating her clitoris with your nose as you move. When she is really wet and aroused and open to receive, gently slide a finger inside her yoni and move it in and out while you continue to stimulate her clitoris with your tongue.

Using your fingers and tongue simultaneously to stimulate her clitoris will create some exquisite sensations for her, and most women enjoy a finger or two in their yoni while it is being kissed. Turn your hand palm up, insert your fingers and crook them slightly, and stroke toward you in a "come hither" motion to hit her G-spot.

The combination of saliva and love juices is considered to have magical properties, which are invigorating and harmonizing for the whole physical system and are to be enjoyed and appreciated. And if you want to get really messy, drip runny honey onto her yoni and lick it off!

LINGAM KISSING

Oral sex is something all men want. The main reasons for this are that there is no pressure and no performance anxiety. It feels good and it is just pure pleasure. When asked what is the most important aspect of lovemaking, most men will say that it's giving pleasure to their lovers. They want to please their lovers and most will often delay the urge to ejaculate. Oral loving gives the man the opportunity to receive and also gives him a visual treat.

A common complaint from men is that women do not perform fellatio often enough, and, perhaps as a result, it is the most popular service performed by prostitutes.

Some women are put off lingam kissing because of the experience of gagging when the lingam is thrust deeply and unexpectedly down their throats. Other women do not like the idea or taste of semen in their mouths. There are ways to deal with both of these responses.

Keeping the mouth and throat relaxed is essential to avoid the gagging reflex. It will increase your pleasure and his. If there is tension or stiffness, you are unable to shield your teeth with your lips and may hurt his lingam. Men seldom, if ever, like to have their lingams bitten—however playfully. The taste of semen varies with diet and

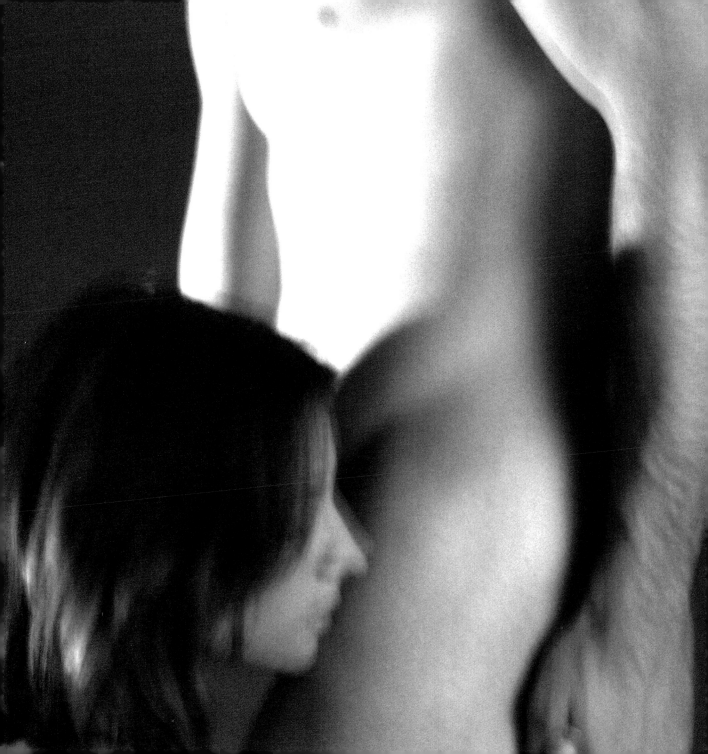

lifestyle. If a man drinks alcohol and coffee and eats meat, the taste of his semen will reflect that. The semen of a vegetarian will taste very different and is said to be the sweetest.

WAYS TO KISS

The optimal position for the lingam kisser is to be facing the man. Try different positions, such as him lying on his back, or him standing and you kneeling or squatting in front of him. Experiment with different scenarios too—get naked but leave him fully clothed with just his zip undone, or stay fully dressed and undress him.

Generally, the greatest thrill for a man is to see his lingam being loved, worshiped, and adored with enthusiasm by his beloved. When you are kissing his lingam, show him that you love doing it. Enthusiasm is the most effective aphrodisiac. Make appreciative noises. Make sure he can see you. A man likes to see your face and watch while you are kissing his lingam. Keep your eyes open and, if you can, hold eye contact.

Give attention to his testicles, perineum, and anus too, before and during. They are all highly erogenous zones. Lick and stroke his perineum, massaging it with light pressure. Gently cradle his testicles in your hand, and lick them or suck them gently, taking one or both in your mouth. Use both hands to stimulate him, one as a guide on his lingam, the other to touch his nipples, testicles, or anus.

The most sensitive area of the lingam is the head, so you can use one hand to hold the shaft while you stimulate the head with your lips and tongue. This technique also gives you more control of how much of his lingam you take into your mouth.

Keep your tongue relaxed (flat) and moist—the wetter the better. The more lubricated your mouth and tongue, the more sensitive and pleasurable it will feel. Do long "lollipop" licks along the shaft, up the side, and around the head. Then cover your teeth with your lips and move up and down the shaft carefully, gently opening and closing your mouth.

When you take his lingam right into your mouth, swirl your tongue around the head and the ridge where the shaft meets the head. Then move it in and out of your mouth with a slow, sucking motion. As his lingam moves in and out of your mouth, slide your (well-lubricated) hand up and down his lingam, closing it when you reach the head and opening it slightly as you slide down the length.

Next, with your lips covering your teeth, encircle his lingam with your mouth so there is a firm and comfortable pressure—a snug fit. Make a gentle twisting motion with your hand as you slide it up and down the shaft, and swirl your tongue around the rim of the head.

Tense your tongue and vibrate it around the head and around the shaft. The more tongue movements while it's in your mouth, the better. Start slowly, keeping a steady rhythm, then increase the pressure and speed up the rhythm.

Take your lover to a peak, staying aware of his body language and his breathing rate, then move your attention to his perineum, testicles, and anus before returning to his lingam.

Experiment with different moves and strokes, such as taking his lingam deeper into your mouth or inserting just the head, or making long slides up and down and alternating with shorter strokes. By doing so, you can both find out what you like doing and what he likes having done to him, and use this knowledge to make your lingam kissing a sublime experience.

If you need to take a break (if your mouth and jaw need a rest), cover your fingers with saliva and slide them across and over the head of his lingam while massaging his scrotum and perineum or prostate with the other hand. If you can use your fingers, lips, and tongue simultaneously he will be thrilled!

VARIOUS TYPES OF LINGAM KISSING AS DESCRIBED IN THE *KAMA SUTRA*

CASUAL
The lingam is held in the hand, placed in the mouth, and moved in between the lips.

NIBBLING THE SIDES
The end of the lingam is covered with one hand, collected together like the bud of a flower. The lips are pressed to the sides and nibble slightly and gently at the same time.

OUTSIDE PRESSING
The lingam is pressed between the lips and kissed as if drawing it out.

INSIDE PRESSING
The lingam is pushed further into the mouth. The lingam is encircled with the partner's lips like a necklace, pressed by the lips and then pulled out.

RUBBING OR BROWSING
After being kissed, the lingam is licked all over with the tip of the tongue, and the tip then passes over its head, titillating the opening.

SUCKING A MANGO
The lingam is put halfway into the mouth and then forcefully kissed and sucked.

SWALLOWING UP OR DEVOURING
The lingam is drawn completely into the mouth, as far as it will go, and then pressed in to the end and sucked, as if being swallowed.

MUTUAL MASTURBATION

Many people do not masturbate regularly once they are past childhood or have become involved in long-term relationships or marriage. And frequently, men and women who do "resort" to masturbation do so with a sense of guilt and shame or a sense of loneliness. For some, the idea of masturbating while in a relationship means there must be something wrong with their sex lives. This is not true! And the benefits of being able to masturbate with your lover or in front of each other are numerous. Psychologically, it deepens intimacy. Through mutual trust, it offers the freedom to be more honest about your feelings. And it increases sexual confidence and self-esteem.

I know that the idea of masturbating in front of your lover is disturbing for some people. This is because they regard masturbation as a deeply personal and private affair. However, if

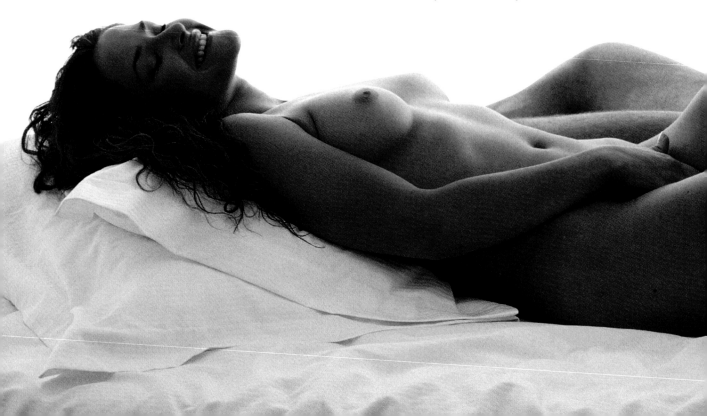

one of you is not in the mood to make love, or when one of you has more sexual desire and energy than the other, the one who is feeling sexual can masturbate while being held by the other, and do so freely and without shame or embarrassment. Often, when one of you is masturbating it can be a turn-on for the other.

"It is for us to learn elsewhere what we are incapable of learning within our own bodies."

SCHWALLER DE LUBICZ

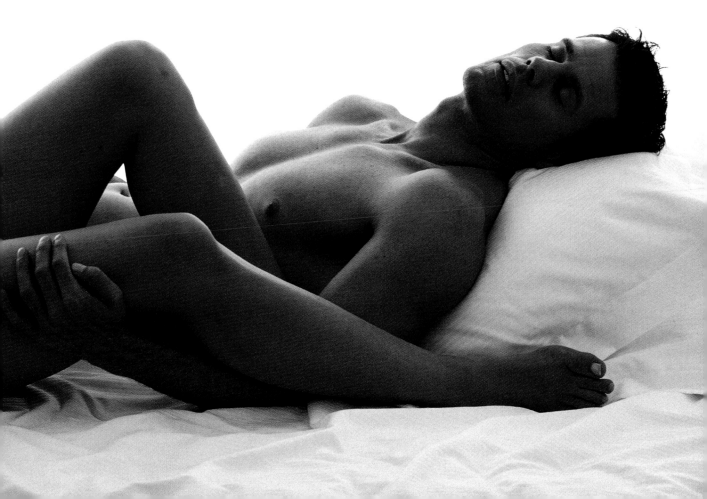

Another benefit of masturbation is that it teaches you a lot about your body's responses to sexual stimulation. And the more in touch you are with your own body, the more attractive you are to your lover.

A GOOD ALTERNATIVE

Intercourse is not the only way to be sexual with one another. The simple act of sharing our self-pleasuring practices with our lovers, wives, or husbands reduces sexual inhibitions, because once we are open enough to masturbate together, we no longer have anything to conceal. This can make sex more fun, and by adding the intimacy of sharing the pleasure of masturbation we give ourselves the opportunity to learn from one another. Watching your lover's techniques and sexual response provides more sexual variety and much more playfulness, which ultimately is the essence of an erotic image of loving.

Sometimes it is even preferable to masturbate rather than have intercourse or oral sex, and it removes any pressure on you to perform sexually. I have occasionally been guilty of starting an argument to create an excuse for avoiding making love. Not very loving or very honest. But not any more!

Of course, there is always the possibility that one of you has reservations about exploring this kind of intimacy. Even the suggestion of it may make your lover feel sexually rejected, or you may fear that if you suggest it, your lover will abandon you because it seems too "kinky." There is also always the possibility that your lover secretly would like to share self-pleasuring, too, but is afraid to ask, convinced the idea would be rejected. So always dare to communicate and share your feelings.

MASTURBATING TOGETHER

Mutual trust, relaxation, and a sense of humor are essential and invaluable assets for this practice. The benefits are that you will feel more at ease with one another, develop mutual respect for one another, and sex will be more fun!

Do whatever it takes to help you relax but don't make orgasm your ultimate goal. Your ultimate goal should be for each of you to find pleasure in your own and your lover's body, and to celebrate your sexual independence together. Do this by showing each other what you do, watching and learning how and where to touch and hold, and observing the different strokes and patterns of movement that give your partner pleasure.

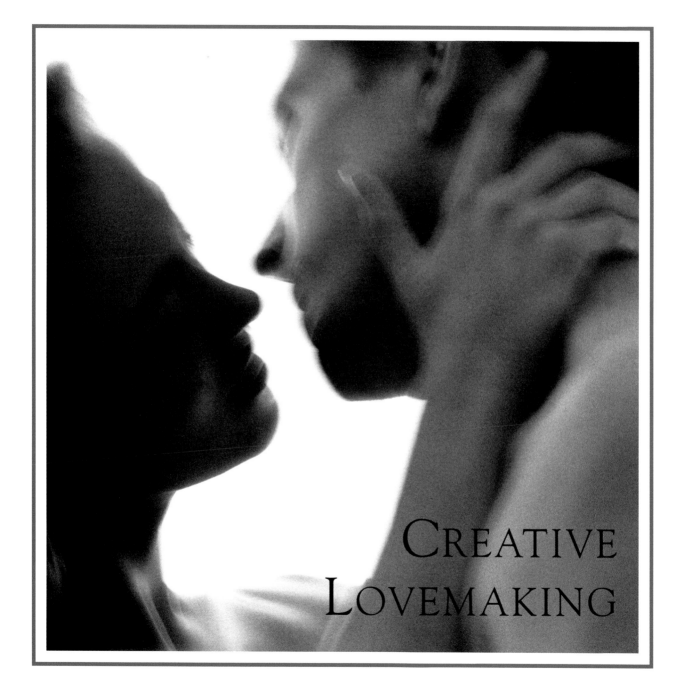

CREATIVE
LOVEMAKING

TAKING THE TIME TO LOVE

"The seed of desire, born of mutual attraction, must develop. To make it grow and flourish much delicacy is needed. It must be watered with the ambrosia of kisses and caresses."

KAMA SUTRA

To make time for making love you need to make your relationship with your lover a priority. It is all too easy to get caught up in the pressures of society and the rush to earn and spend, and to become so distracted that you start to neglect one of the most precious things in your life—your lover. We want it all and we want it now—from instant coffee to fast food to instant love. If we put as much energy into our relationships as we do into other activities, how different our experience of life would be.

Just as you need to make time to be with your lover, so you need to take time loving your lover. Vatsyayana, author of the *Kama Sutra*, draws attention to the fact that if a man gets too carried away by his own excitation at the beginning of lovemaking, the woman will not experience pleasure. He reminds us that women are not only fragile in their limbs, but also in their

feelings and minds. He recommends that a man should consider a woman to be like a flower. He must treat her in such a way that she will not close up, but will open out and diffuse her scent. She must be treated with an understanding of her state of mind and fragility. With patience and sweetness, the man must drive away the woman's natural apprehensions.

Men and women are different, and experience lovemaking differently. For a man, sexual union happens outside his body; for a woman, sexual union takes place inside her body. The emphasis on the importance of the female orgasm has tended to detract from the woman's equally important need for emotional satisfaction from sex—for tenderness, love, admiration, close communion, and intimacy. The same is true for men, who are often portrayed or expected to respond like sexual machines instead of human beings. Whether you are a man or a woman; each of us holds elements of the masculine and feminine within us in varying degrees and at different times. Despite their differences, what men and women want from one another in love is very similar, and for both men and women the greatest joy is in the giving.

What Women Want

What a woman wants is to be treated and cherished like a goddess. A woman wants to feel attractive and to be accepted and loved just the way she is. A woman wants her lover to care, and to want to please and satisfy her sexually. She wants her lover to discover and appreciate all of her body and to know where and how to touch her and to ask her what she likes and dislikes. She wants her lover to be open to her and for her to be able to say openly what she wants, and for it to be fine for her to say so. She wants her toes to be considered as important as her nipples. A woman wants to feel that she excites and turns her lover on.

A woman also likes a build-up to lovemaking, whether it is going out for the evening or spending time touching and caressing as a kind of foreplay. She wants to take time over lovemaking, without hurrying it, although a "quickie" can sometimes be very erotic. She wants to be playful. And what she wants most of all is to feel her lover's total presence, fully focused. She also wants to feel her lover's intelligence, strength, passion, direction, and humor.

What Men Want

Apart from a lover who is great in bed, a man wants sexual openness, trust, support, intelligence, sensitivity, intimacy, and the space to be vulnerable. He also wants to give his lover pleasure and to

"For a man as for a woman, the total gift of self is a source of wonderful happiness and luck. Sexual intercourse is not merely a pleasure of the senses: more important is the sacrifice of oneself, the gift of self."

KAMA SUTRA

feel her receiving it. He wants to see her pleasure reflected in how she moves, moans, smiles, and opens herself to welcome him in. A man needs to be encouraged with words and sounds.

A woman's energy, responsiveness and sexual delight are enchanting to a man. He wants to be turned on by her total ecstatic surrender. When a man sees a woman enjoying her femininity, he becomes absorbed in the radiance of her happiness and her pleasure.

LOVE POSITIONS

Using different lovemaking positions offers variety, helps to prolong intercourse, and can provide healing. On the following pages I describe some old, some new, some familiar, and some forgotten positions, all tried and tested over thousands of years by millions of people. Think of these positions as suggestions to help you find the ones that suit you best.

Different positions will be better for certain styles and types of thrusting. And some positions will work better for you than others, depending on the shape, height, and weight of your body and the placement, depth, width, and length of your genitals.

Enjoy the discovery of searching for the best positions for you and your lover, and keep the interest and zest for making love with one another refreshing and alive. Adapt the positions described here to your own needs in an imaginative way—there's no need to copy them exactly. It's also fun to make up your own names for the postures you experiment with, too. It introduces an element of humor, which is always welcome in lovemaking.

Experimenting with lovemaking positions is important because we are all guilty, especially in long-term relationships, of restricting ourselves to a few familiar positions that we know work well for us. However, monotony can be dangerous because it leads to boredom and then sex becomes a mechanical exercise.

EASY VARIATIONS

If you are not feeling particularly adventurous, even a slight change—the use of a pillow or cushion, or a realignment of the legs—allows you the opportunity of experiencing new sensations. This works by varying the angle of the yoni relative to the lingam, and is particularly effective in positions where the woman lies on her back.

In such a position, placing a cushion under her pelvic region, roughly between the small of her back and the base of her spine, makes the position of the yoni curve downward and outward. Intercourse in this position brings the lingam in contact with the clitoris and allows for deep penetration. Similarly, putting a cushion just below and under her buttocks makes the angle of her yoni curve upward and inward so that the yoni canal lies at roughly the same angle as the lingam. This leads to a satisfyingly deep penetration with the possibility of intense orgasm.

Give yourself time to savor a variety of positions and thrusts, because even a slight change in the relative positions of your two bodies is enough to vary the sensations you experience. And if you ring the changes in your positions, techniques, and skills, you will not need to ring the changes in your lover.

The four basic positions of lovemaking are man on top, woman on top, man behind, and side-by-side in sitting or kneeling positions. There are also the lesser-practiced standing positions. All these positions have endless variations. Some create a stimulating and positive type of sexual tension while others are more peaceful, allowing a couple to stay together in union without having to move, which affords a different kind of intimacy.

Some of these postures are a clear indication why fitness and agility are vitally important. Many yoga postures reflect different love positions and serve as preparation for adventurous lovemaking. Please remember: if a particular position is creating physical strain or is painful, do not continue it.

All the movements of intercourse and lovemaking should be done with grace and coordination. And there is particular satisfaction to be gained from moving from one position to another without having to withdraw the lingam from the yoni, with the minimum of movements and with the greatest harmony between the couple.

WOMAN ON TOP

The advantage of these positions is that the woman takes an active role and can select for herself the most exciting approach and angle of thrusting. Some women find this the best position for reaching orgasm. The advantage for the man is that if he has been proactive, he gets a break to relax and enjoy himself. He also gets the pleasure of seeing his lover on top while still having easy access to her breasts and the rest of her body.

In this position, some men find it easier to control ejaculation. It can also

A woman-on top position lets the woman control the speed and depth of the thrusting. This often makes it easier for the man to relax and control his ejaculation.

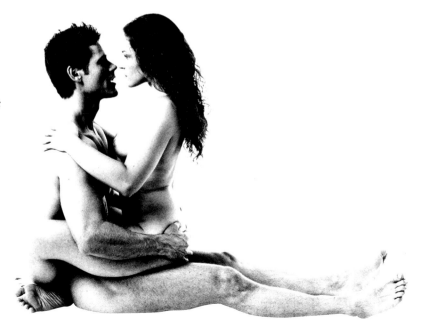

be a useful position if the man is very much heavier than the woman or if he is tired. Another good time for couples to use it is when they want to make love during the first few months of pregnancy—the woman has no weight on her in this position.

THE SNAKE POSTURE

Facing her lover, the woman gradually lowers herself onto his lingam, with her legs either inside or outside his. She can either bend her knees or put her feet flat either side of her lover. If she puts her legs inside her lover's, she can squeeze his lingam gently with her thighs and so encourage erection. Her lover can caress her breasts and nipples and increase her arousal.

PAIR OF TONGS

To get into this position, the man sits down with his hands behind him, to take the weight. The woman crouches over her lover and gently lowers herself onto his lingam. Then she brings her legs forward and wraps them around him so that he can sit up properly. In a variation on this position, the woman leans back along his legs and takes her weight on her elbows.

GEESE FLYING ON THEIR BACKS

This position usually begins with the woman sitting on top of her lover, facing him with his lingam inside her. She then turns 180 degrees—which can be very stimulating for his lingam—so that she is now facing his feet with her hands resting on his ankles. She can produce variations in the sensations she feels by leaning forward and changing the angle of penetration. If she wishes, she can gradually lower her head until her face is on the sheets between her lover's legs. He can either sit up slightly or lie down flat on his back and fondle her buttocks and clitoris.

REVERSED FLYING DUCKS

This position is excellent for slow and prolonged lovemaking and it lets the woman control penetration. It is also a good position if the man is much heavier than the woman, or if she is pregnant, as she does not have to bear his weight.

To get into the position, he sits on the bed, leaning on his elbows with his legs straight out in front of him. She then kneels with her back to him, her legs either side of his. The woman can increase her own pleasure by making circular movements with her hips.

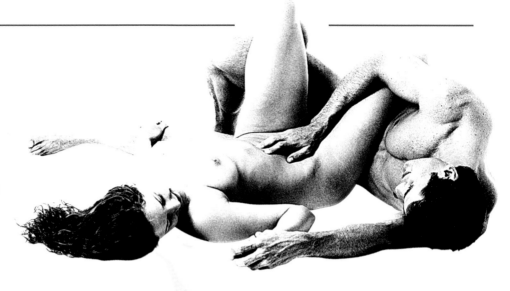

SIDE-BY-SIDE

Side-by-side positions are comfortable and allow the couple to regulate the depth of penetration. They also are very useful when the woman is pregnant because lovemaking can continue when her belly starts to get in the way of more conventional positions.

MANDARIN DUCKS

This position is good for gentle lovemaking, with slow unhurried movements. This is also a good position for the first months of pregnancy.

Lying on her side, and tilted slightly backward to avoid taking the full weight of her lover on her lower leg, the woman draws both legs up above her lover's hips. With her legs around her lover they are comfortably wide apart, exposing her entire yoni for complete penetration as well as maximum stimulation by the lingam.

THE CRAB

This is a good position for energetic, passionate lovemaking in a close, intimate embrace. The couple lie facing each other, then the woman hooks one leg over her lover's body while swiveling her hips slightly toward him and keeping her other leg straight. He does the same, lower down, so that he can penetrate his lover easily and thrust rhythmically. Because her head will be slightly above his, this is an excellent position for the man to give his partner plenty of breast and nipple stimulation. At the same time, the woman can fondle his buttocks and thighs.

THE CARRIAGE POSTURE

In this position the woman lies flat on her back with her knees bent. Her lover lies on his side with the lower part of his body under her bottom so that her legs go across his thighs. This position gives the lovers the opportunity to look into each other's eyes and to caress and embrace each other.

The Carriage Posture allows lovers to look into each other's eyes and to touch, caress, and embrace each other.

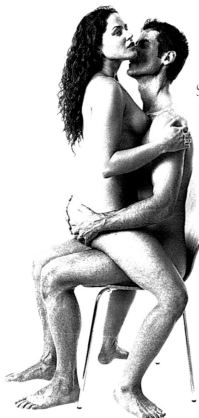

In the Seated Lotus position, the woman creates and controls the thrusting action by moving up and down on her feet.

SITTING

Sitting positions are wonderful for covert lovemaking while dressed, and the thrill of a clandestine experience adds a different dimension to lovemaking. Sitting positions can be less easy to move in, but, there are some advantages to that. They help you to prolong lovemaking or just to experience the physical closeness of one another.

SEATED LOTUS

With the man sitting on a chair, his lover can straddle him facing him, and if she can reach the floor she can move up and down on her feet. Or she can sit on his lap facing away from him, while he embraces her belly and stimulates her breasts and clitoris.

SPLITTING THE BAMBOO

Another variation is for the woman to sit on her lover's lap, turn sideways, and raise the leg that is next to her lover's body. This position allows deep penetration, simultaneous manual stimulation of breasts and clitoris, and passionate mouth-to-mouth kissing.

THE PAIRED FEET POSITION

In this position, the man sits on the bed with his legs outstretched and apart. Facing him, the woman lowers herself onto his lingam and leans back, taking her weight on her elbows, then she raises her knees and he gently squeezes her thighs together. This position restricts the movements of both lovers and reduces the amount of genital stimulation, which makes it a good position if you want to "calm down" and prolong your lovemaking.

REAR ENTRY

These positions are not a form of anal intercourse, simply those in which the man approaches the woman from behind. Rear-entry positions are animal-like and create a strong feeling of primitive sexuality. The man can thrust deeply and slowly, while his hands are free to stimulate his partner's breasts and clitoris.

When you are making love in any of the rear-entry positions, the man should always begin with gentle thrusting and build up slowly to more vigorous action. He should not thrust too vigorously too soon because it might cause his lover discomfort if she is not fully aroused.

JUMPING WHITE TIGER

The woman kneels on her hands and knees. The man kneels behind her and can stimulate her clitoris and breasts.

DARK CICADA FIXED TO A TREE

In this variation on the Jumping White Tiger, the woman kneels and inclines her body forward, resting her head on her folded arms while the man kneels behind her. He holds his lover's hips and urges himself into her. This position thrusts the yoni upward and allows the lingam to enter with ease.

It is probably worth mentioning that in this position, as the man thrusts in and out, the woman's yoni may emit a sound because of the escaping air. But don't let it put you off. Once you have got over the possible initial surprise and embarrassment, enjoy the sound as an erotic addition—even a humorous one!

REVERSED BEE BUZZING OVER MAN

You can also enjoy rear-entry lovemaking with the man lying on his back. In this position, the man lies on his back with his legs straight out in front, either together or slightly apart. The woman kneels over him with her back to him, so that she is squatting astride him. She can move her pelvis up and down and from side to side in this position while fondling her lover's testicles. He can massage her shoulders, back, buttocks, or thighs, and to vary the sensations he can raise himself by gripping her shoulders or hips.

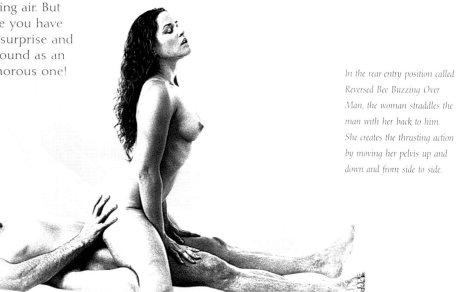

In the rear-entry position called Reversed Bee Buzzing Over Man, the woman straddles the man with her back to him. She creates the thrusting action by moving her pelvis up and down and from side to side.

DONKEYS IN THE THIRD MOON OF SPRING

Both lovers need to be fit and agile to use the Donkeys in the Third Moon of Spring position, but it can be very satisfying because the man can thrust slowly and deeply.

This rear-entry position is for the agile. The woman lies face-down on the bed with her legs apart and hanging over the edge. The man stands or kneels between her legs, and, as she raises her hips, he bends down to gently grasp her thighs, lifting her legs up in the air rather like in a child's wheelbarrow game. As she hangs her head and rests on her elbows, he can rhythmically thrust slowly and deeply. The woman can either lie with her legs held straight or hook them around her lover's back.

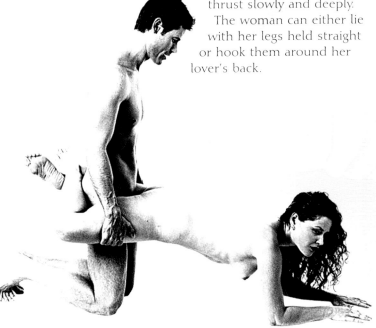

STANDING POSITIONS

Making love standing requires both lovers to stay in the moment in order to maintain their balance, and can be an enjoyable addition to your repertoire.

BASIC STANDING POSITION

The basic standing position is much easier if you and your lover are about the same height, otherwise the taller of you will have to bend his or her knees to maintain penetration. It is best performed leaning against a wall or other back-support to give thrusting more vigor. It is a good position for caressing each other as well as for prolonged, passionate kissing.

THE SUSPENDED POSITION

A more adventurous variation is when the man holds the woman and completely supports her weight. To begin, it helps if the woman sits on a high stool or counter top of the right height. Her lover clasps her tightly in his arms while she wraps her legs around his back, and gradually he lifts her off her seat until he is holding her right off the floor. He can hold her in position by gripping her under her buttocks.

One drawback of this position is that thrusting is difficult. But on the plus side, it offers deep penetration and a thrilling sense of closeness.

THREE STEPS OF VISHNU

For this next posture it helps to be fit, and you will most likely need the support of a wall behind you. Move into this position slowly and carefully to avoid straining any back or leg muscles.

The couple prepare to get into the position by standing facing each other. The man then puts his hand under his lover's buttocks to support her while she wraps her left leg over his right thigh. He then penetrates her yoni with his lingam and wraps his left leg around her right thigh.

STEPPING BEYOND

This posture may require some practice and adaptation, and it is important that both partners are flexible and strong.

The woman lies on her back with her legs apart while the man stands diagonally across her. Bracing herself on her arms, she then pushes herself up onto her shoulders and raises one leg, taking her weight on her other leg. The man can help by holding her raised leg and gently pulling her upward.

Once in this position, the man lowers himself into the woman and thrusts by rocking from foot to foot. If the man is worried about losing his balance standing on a bed, try this on the floor with the woman's head and shoulders resting on cushions and pillows to ensure she is comfortable.

MAN ON TOP

The basic man-on-top lovemaking posture is known as the missionary position. Most of the variations on this involve the woman changing the positions of her legs to vary the sensations both partners feel.

OPENING AND BLOSSOMING

This is an intimate lovemaking position. The woman lies on her back with her knees drawn up to her chest. Her lover kneels with his thighs on either side of her hips and enters her. She then hooks her legs over his arms and he eases them onto his shoulders.

Making love in this position involves deep penetration, so extended loveplay may be necessary to help the woman relax enough to be able to enjoy it. In this position the man can lovingly caress her breasts and legs and use his hands to give additional clitoral stimulation. It is important that he enters her gently and thrusts slowly to start with. As the excitement increases, he can gain additional thrust by holding her and pulling her toward him.

EQUAL LEGGED

This position requires the woman to be both fit and flexible. To start off, she lies flat on her back and her lover kneels between her legs. Then she draws her legs back, lifts them up, places the backs of her calves on his shoulders, and carefully hooks her legs around the back of his neck.

This position allows very deep penetration, so it is essential that the man enters the woman very carefully and gently. The position is probably easiest to use after the couple have spent some time making love. By then, the woman's muscles will have relaxed, making it easier to get into the position, and she will be well-lubricated so penetration will be easier.

TENSION POSITIONS

Intended to be stimulating, tension positions build up arousal while maintaining feelings of closeness and calmness. When you're using one of these positions, you may want to hold the position or move with tantalizing and exquisite slowness.

COBRA

The woman sits astride the man facing him with her knees on the bed, then arches her back as far back as she can and holds onto his ankles, if possible.

THE LOVE RACK

With either the man or the woman on top, both stretch your arms and legs out as far as you can.

THE PENETRATOR

With the man on top and a wall at his feet, he slowly penetrates and presses powerfully into her while pressing his feet against the wall behind him.

ELIXIR

An interesting variation on the missionary position is for the woman to draw her legs back until her knees are near her ears. This raises the position of her yoni and it gives a depth of penetration difficult to achieve in other positions. Unless she is very flexible, the woman will need to hold her legs with her hands. The man will have to crouch in order to maintain contact in this position, but the depth of penetration gives a feeling of closeness that makes this position worth trying, even briefly.

You won't be able to hold this position comfortably for too long because of the pressure on the woman's abdomen. So it is advisable not to do it after eating a big meal!

THE BOW

It is easy to move into this position from the Elixir position—the woman lowers her legs and places them on the man's shoulders. He may need to raise himself to support himself on his hands and toes, so his body is positioned in a straight incline over hers and making only genital contact.

Lowering her legs still further, the woman crosses her legs over the man's hips and uses the power of her leg muscles to lock the sexual embrace. This position shortens the yoni and the man's lingam is likely to touch the cervix, so proceed with care.

Your movements will be restricted when you are in this position, so use it as an opportunity to breathe together and gaze into each other's eyes.

ROARING

In this position, the woman lies with the base of her spine at the very edge of the bed, with legs apart. The man faces her and kneels on the floor, either on one or both knees. He gently penetrates her and then she sits up, supported by

his embrace, and hooks her legs behind his back.

This position is an especially good one for combining loveplay with intercourse. It allows you to kiss and to caress each other with your hands, and allows deep penetration combined with clitoral stimulation.

PLEASANT VARIATIONS

In most lovemaking positions, the man is positioned between the woman's legs. For a variation of sensations when you're using such a position, reverse the situation so that the man's legs are placed outside the woman's.

To enhance the yoni's grasp on the lingam during penetration when the man's legs are outside hers, the woman

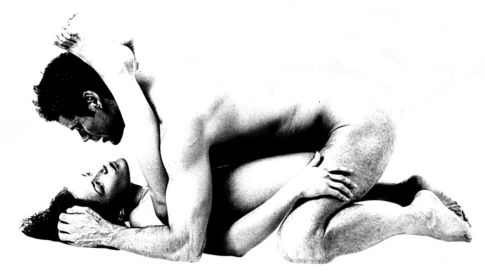

The Elixir position is difficult to maintain for long, but it gives an incredible depth of penetration and a wonderful feeling of closeness.

should cross her legs at knee-level. When she does this, her closed-up yoni walls will tighten around the base of his lingam, restricting its movement and ensuring the closest possible contact between lingam and yoni. And in this position, both the man and the woman can practice their PC muscle clenches and releases.

PEACEFUL POSITIONS

These positions give restful intercourse with a minimum of movement for both the man and the woman.

They also help you to prolong intercourse by taking a break from the more active positions. This gives you time to absorb the sexual energy you have already created.

There is great value and fulfillment in taking time to be still with one another and to appreciate the sight, sounds, smell, and touch sensations of staying together without moving. It slows down your minds, keeps you present with one another, and offers an opportunity for maintaining eye contact.

To relax and experience inner peace and contentment in this way is a sexual love meditation.

ENTWINED CLASPING

The man lies on the right of the woman, lying on his left side and facing her. Lying on her right side, she places her right leg in between his legs and her left leg on top of them.

When a couple are in this position, the interlacing of their legs ensures that genital contact will be maintained easily. This is a comfortable position for slow, sensual intercourse and also a lovely one to fall asleep in together.

YAB YUM

This is the classic position of Tantric iconography. Most Tantric deities are depicted in close sexual embrace with their Shaktis (goddesses) in the Yab Yum posture. It indicates the power of sex, the strength of the union, and the dependence of the male principle on the female and vice versa.

It is an easy position to move into from the missionary position or the basic woman-on-top position. The man sits with his legs crossed or slightly bent, and the soles of his feet touching. The woman sits on top of him, facing him with her legs crossed behind his back and her arms embracing him around his back or around his neck. The man can place his hands under her buttocks and move, or the man and woman can simply stay completely still, gazing into each other's eyes, breathing together, and even practicing clenching and releasing the PC muscles. However, penetration involving deep movement is restricted.

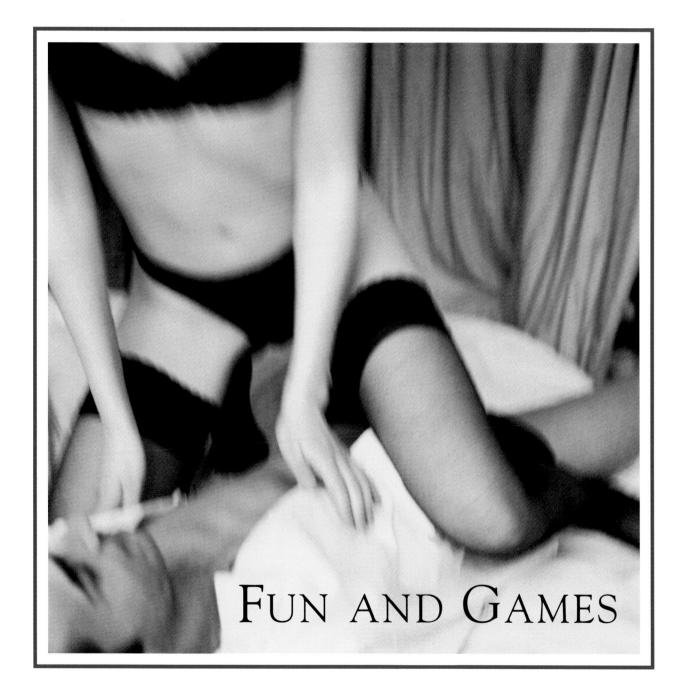

FUN AND GAMES

FANTASY

"Developing new fantasies is about exploring our minds and emotions for sexual content that will enhance our enjoyment of orgasms. As we learn to have more creative sex lives alone and with our lovers, maybe we will also become more generous about sharing the rich details of our fantasy worlds. Playing the game 'I'll tell you mine if you tell me yours' we could inspire one another in our pursuit of sexual happiness."

BETTY DODSON

Sexual fantasy is a normal, natural activity and an integral part of our sexuality. And, as yet, no one can read our minds!

When your lover is enjoying erotic fantasies, it does not mean that he or she is betraying you or that the love he or she has for you is inadequate. Fantasizing about something does not necessarily mean you will actually do it—a lot of us imagine things we never intend to experience.

The beauty of fantasy is that it allows you the freedom to experiment with sexual variety beyond the limits of reality. By using your creative mind, you open up endless possibilities that can exist far beyond the restrictions of reality. Fantasies also can help you to focus your body and mind and the sensations they produce.

There is no such thing as an abnormal fantasy as long as you can distinguish between it and reality, and there is no need to pass judgment on your sexual imagination. Honor your fantasies and your ability to fantasize, but do not mistake them for reality.

It is true that sexual fantasies, private or shared, have probably always been used to make sex more exciting. Or where, for whatever reason, sex has been impossible, fantasies have proved to be good substitutes or helped to fill a hopeless void! They can provide escape from the mundane, may promote heightened pleasure, or be truly revelatory as well as an essential means of sexual self-discovery.

Some people find it much easier to fantasize than others, however it is something that you can teach yourself

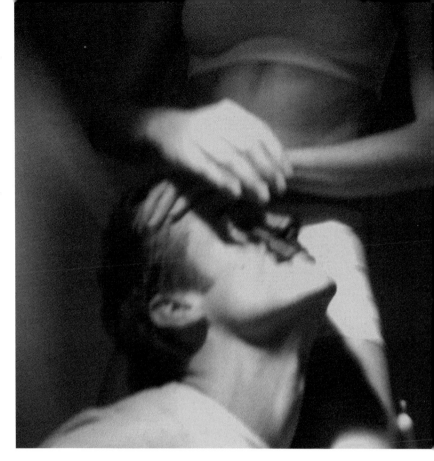

to do. What you need is to feel comfortable enough with your sexual thoughts to let go, to feel good about yourself, and to be willing to trust yourself and a free and rich imagination. Sexual fantasy is not a large part of some women's lives, though romantic love stories with huge emotional content are. If you are one of these women, you could experiment by masturbating while looking at erotic literature or a sexy film.

The largest sex organ of the body is the brain, and our minds and our imaginations provide us with the most effective of all aphrodisiacs. Erotic fantasies link our conscious and subconscious minds, allowing us to explore our sexuality and give play to our creative souls. Fantasies make the forbidden, the foolish, and the wild all accessible. They can be funny, somber, daring, scary, wicked, and raunchy, and there is the possibility that in the process of exploration, some surprising and unexpected sexual situations will appear from the deep recesses of our unconscious minds.

Dreams and daydreams are all forms of fantasy. Some fantasies are based on real-life situations while others have a more mythical or mystical nature, even other-cultural. A common theme of a lot of fantasies is an erotic tension—the play between seeming opposites. These opposites include inhibition and abandon, freedom and the forbidden, power and submission, safety and exploration, and fantasy and reality.

Fantasies can be based on an idea, an image, a sound, or a vague feeling, and developed and expanded into an imaginary world or scene. The stronger your fantasy life and visualizations, the easier it will be to increase your arousal when you wish—alone or together with your lover.

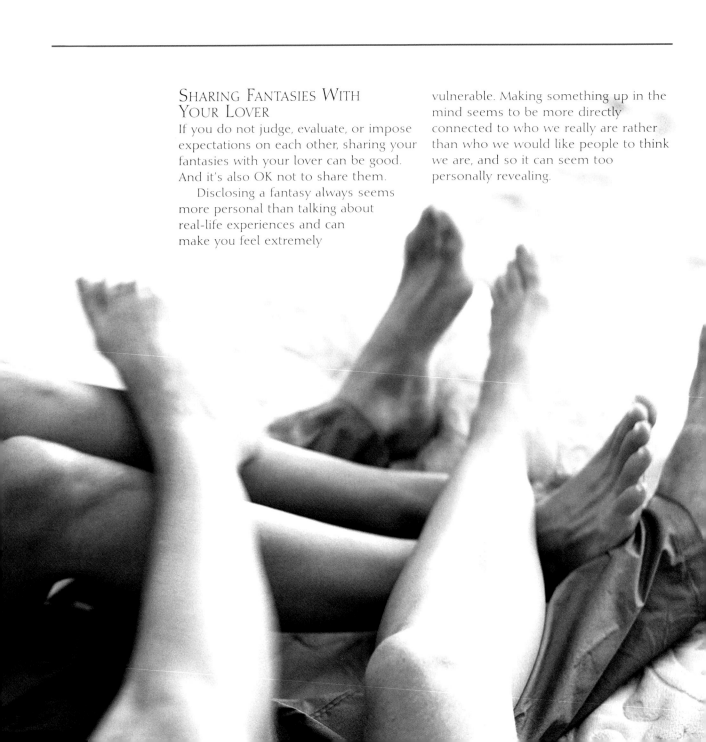

SHARING FANTASIES WITH YOUR LOVER

If you do not judge, evaluate, or impose expectations on each other, sharing your fantasies with your lover can be good. And it's also OK not to share them.

Disclosing a fantasy always seems more personal than talking about real-life experiences and can make you feel extremely vulnerable. Making something up in the mind seems to be more directly connected to who we really are rather than who we would like people to think we are, and so it can seem too personally revealing.

Acting out a sexual fantasy with a lover requires honest communication and willing consent. Choose fantasies that appeal to both of you and work out the scenario together beforehand.

My lover and I once decided to spice up our love life and act out a fantasy that I was a prostitute and he a client. He went out while I prepared myself. I dressed up in stockings and high heels. We arranged a time when he would return, and we would greet each other as strangers and then seduce one another. We did not plan any more than that, and we remember feeling slightly awkward and unsure of ourselves before breaking down in fits of giggles. Mutual consent and a sense of humor are of the utmost importance!

Positive creative fantasies and visualizations can be an important ingredient of masturbation and creating intimacy when you both consent to act them out, as long as they cause no harm to yourselves or to others. Do not be tempted to fantasize about someone other than your lover when you are making love. You need to be emotionally and spiritually present with your lover when making love, so you are not distracted from the exchanges of energy and the subtle blending of each other's sexual energies.

The danger of relying on sexual fantasy is that sex will become limited to a mind trip. If sex becomes a mental play, it can take you out of your feeling body. It can block the deepest part of your being because it is not centered in your body in the present moment but in projecting ahead into the future.

The Taoists believe that if your mind is concentrating on something different from what the body is doing, it creates a rift between the mental and spiritual aspects of your body. So when you make love, your thoughts must be on lovemaking and on feeling love.

MAKING LOVE WITH A GOD OR GODDESS

In Tantra, visualization is used to raise the consciousness of lovemaking to a sacred act. As a way of elevating your sexual love to a higher plane, you can visualize your beloved as a god or goddess, worship the divinity within each other, and experience the sacredness of sex. By cultivating your lover as a divine image, you promote feelings in your heart of reverence, awe, high esteem, deep respect, and humility.

When a god and goddess make love, the experience is uplifting. And cosmic role-playing is fun, too; it is an opportunity to express a different aspect of yourselves. You can give each other unusual, ethereal names, drape yourselves with sensual fabrics, adorn each other with exotic accessories, and with lighting and music create the ideal setting to free your erotic imagination.

GAMES LOVERS CAN PLAY

"We don't stop playing because we grow old; we grow old because we stop playing."

GEORGE BERNARD SHAW

When your sex life and/or love life are important enough to you to invest time and energy into them, experiment with some or all of these suggestions of things to do together with your lover. It will help if you keep hold of your sense of humor and don't shy away from some healthy self-observation, which some of the suggestions are bound to evoke. If nothing else, this will give you both something to talk about or inspire you to create your own amusements!

Some of the following are Tantric sexual instructions of the *Ragamaya*, others I have made up, and, dare I say, even tried!

- Breathing slowly together and looking into each other's eyes, contemplate the other as love, energy, or the void.
- Assume playful roles, with or without dressing up, and make love in the roles. Try switching genders.
- Blindfold your lover and ask sexually explicit questions or get him or her to explore your body while you watch.

- Get dressed and strip for one another.
- Go to sleep together and set the alarm for the middle of the night. As soon as the alarm rings, reach for your lover and begin to make love to him or her.
- As you make love, invent spontaneous names for the erotic parts of your lover's body—breasts, mouth, vagina, penis. Say them out loud: "I want to lick your shnnogily, I want to nibble your nipalickolop."
- With a green felt-tipped pen, place a dot on the center of your lover's chest or in the center of his or her forehead (the third eye) or anywhere else on your lover's body. Concentrate on that mark the whole time you make love.
- Imagine your body is made of stone and very heavy so every movement and gesture takes great concentration.
- Imagine your body is very light; concentrate on not floating away.
- Dance together; dance for each other; dance naked and celebrate!
- Put on a hat or a beautiful piece of jewelry and nothing else.

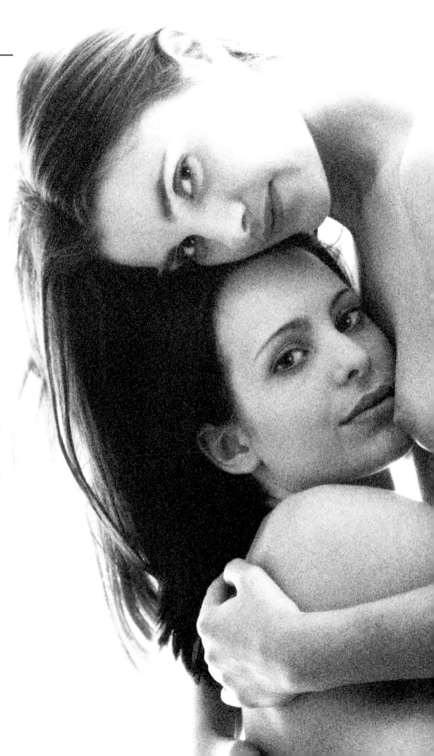

- Choose your favorite animals and make love like those animals.
- Keep eye contact with your lover the entire time you are making love.
- Using an instant picture camera, take sexy and erotic pictures of one another; or film yourselves together doing whatever!
- The next time you make love, one of you do absolutely nothing.
- Have a playful pillow fight and yell and scream until you are exhausted, then make love.
- Write down, text, or e-mail something you want your lover to do that he or she has never done before, perhaps something that is a dream or fantasy of yours.
- Lie down next to each other, eyes closed. Without physical contact make love in your minds.
- Make love as though it was the first time for both of you or as if this were the very last time.
- Shave each other's pubic hair in a design or completely naked.
- Some time when you really don't want to make love, do it. Some time when you really do want to make love, don't.
- Dress up in each other's clothes. Then make love role playing each other.
- Sit facing each other each with a bowl of favorite foods or fruit. Act as if you are making love with each other, only

do it with the food or fruit and do not touch one another.

- Undress one another with your hands behind your backs.
- Use a clean, soft, thick paintbrush and paint your lover's body with something edible.
- If you can, experience sleeping in one bed and making love in another.
- Tell each other an erotic story by taking it in turns to make up and tell each part of it.
- Surprise your lover in some way.
- Slip a sexy note into your lover's pocket or purse.
  - Eat a meal together using only your hands. Use your fingers to feed one another.
    - Play the mirror game. To do this, you stand face-to-face and one of you mirrors exactly what the other is doing, whether it is a movement, sound, gesture, expression, or physical act. This game helps you both to break down any selfconsciousness you might feel. It also allows each of you to play out different roles and express different attitudes, which allows an intimacy and harmonization in unspoken communication. And it's fun!
- Make a ritual of your lovemaking. Prepare the space, anoint each other with oils, light candles and incense, and honor one another as a god or goddess. Make love as an act of mutual worship.
- Use game-playing to have fun with one another and to explore different aspects of yourselves. They are an opportunity to let go of inhibitions and to give the love you have to give.

PORNOGRAPHY AND EROTICA

"The difference between pornography and erotica is lighting."

GLORIA LEONARD

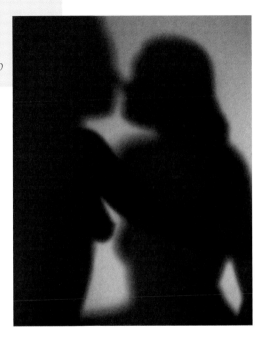

Our interest in reading sexually explicit materials or in looking at pictures of sexual acts or organs is hardly new. Every civilization has created its own erotica, as though it were a fundamental form of human expression and a manifestation of the fantasy element of human sexuality.

Illustrated sex manuals and pillow books have played an important part in Eastern cultures from the earliest days, and there is plenty of extant erotic art from ancient civilizations in Africa and the Middle East. Down the centuries, books about sex have been widely and eagerly read for both educational and entertainment purposes.

Pornography and erotica are much used as sex aids. The distinction between the two is rather blurred and depends to some extent on individual judgment. Basically, pornography is concerned with just the physical act of sex or depicting genitals in a straightforward way, while erotica is more an attempt to portray love in its physical manifestations. Material intended to arouse is as varied as the people it arouses and there is a place for both as sex aids.

Most people find pornography exciting at times, although some people have been conditioned into being reluctant to admit it openly. At other times, they may find pornography so crude as to be quite offensive. On the other hand, the subtlety of erotica can be very inspiring and arousing, and a real help in finding sexual excitement. People are more likely to be sexually aroused by content to which they can relate, rather than by portrayals of sexual acts that they find uncomfortable or offensive. However, it does depend on your mood.

All pornography is about sex and, until fairly recently, "adult entertainment" was a male-dominated industry created by and aimed at male desire and inclination. In the past, it was generally assumed that men responded more powerfully to erotic material than women did. However, research indicates that this is not the case: both sexes respond to pornography and erotica in similar ways, although the male usually has more obvious external evidence of his arousal!

Adult films created, produced, and directed by women, exploring what women desire and want from sex, are now more available and increasingly popular. Such films tend to have a softer, more sensual, and more erotic approach, and they tend to attract an ever-growing segment of society— women eager to explore their own fantasies. Such women are seeking sexually fulfilling experiences and are eager to find new and fun ways of sharing a sexy evening with a lover!

Pornography flourishes because there are many reasons why people use it. Pornography and erotica provide a source of knowledge and comparative information about sexual behavior. They can be a substitute for sex for people who don't have or want a lover, or who see it as more pleasurable and less bother than other options. It can also be a means of arousing oneself or a lover, a welcome aphrodisiac.

Using Porn for Pleasure

If your lover uses porn occasionally, it doesn't mean that love has gone or that you are or have become inadequate. People use pornography and erotica to accompany masturbation and to stimulate sexual desire. Some people use it during sex to add a different dimension. I know of a number of couples in long-standing relationships where, for a variety of reasons, the sex has diminished somewhat, who have found that watching pornography together has imbued their sex lives with a renewed source of energy.

If you use porn as a sex aid, just be sensitive about it. It can inspire and excite at the right time; it also can upset your lover if it clashes with the feelings of the moment. If you are obsessed with porn and unable to enjoy sex with your lover, that may be something you need to address.

SEX TOYS

The fact that love instruments, implements, and devices (or sex aids) have been around for centuries is perhaps historical proof that seeking sexual satisfaction is a basic human desire.

Mentioned in the *Kama Sutra* and in a number of other Indian and Chinese texts, love instruments were, and are still, used to augment or substitute for the sexual organs. Phalluses carved from exquisite woods, or made of ivory, horn, or jade, or even cast in gold and silver, have been found in nearly every culture. Some were ancient religious symbols of fertility, some were used to ward off evil or to bring luck, and others were designed purely for the pleasure of both men and women.

MALE ACCOUTREMENTS

Various devices to be put on or over the lingam to supplement its length or thickness are frequently described in Asian literature and ancient texts.

There also are accounts of special rings, often made of jade, that fitted around the base of the lingam. These had small protruding parts that were used to stimulate the woman's clitoris during lovemaking. These ancient devices were the forerunners of the modern cock ring.

FEMALE IMPLEMENTS

There are also ancient references to the double dildo, a device with two silk bands attached in the middle. One woman could insert one end into her own yoni, fastening it with ribbons tied around her waist. Then she could satisfy the other woman with the prominent end of the shaft, while herself enjoying the friction produced from the movement of the other end inside her. Another Oriental innovation, commonly known as "Ben-Wa Balls," consisted of a pair of hollow spheres made of silver, one containing a drop of mercury, which were inserted into the yoni so that as the woman moved, they created a gentle vibration inside her.

VIBRATORS AND DILDOS

Vibrators are electric massagers (usually battery-powered) that may be used for internal or external stimulation. Dildos are designed for either vaginal or anal insertion, and, generally, do not vibrate. Those that do are usually called "vibrating dildos."

Dildos create a satisfying sensation of internal fullness and pressure, which many women and men find highly pleasurable. Dildos are the perfect option if you require something to use for penetration, while a vibrator is more

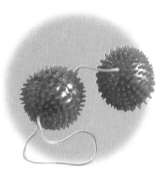
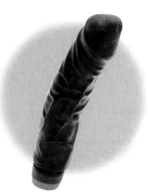
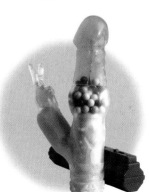

appropriate if you are looking for something that provides arousing clitoral stimulation.

The first vibrator was probably the steam-powered massage and vibratory apparatus patented in 1869 by Dr. George Taylor, an American physician, for treatment of female disorders. The medical treatment for women suffering from "hysteria" at that time was to manually stimulate their genitals until they reached orgasm (known as "hysterical paroxysm"). The first vibrator made the stimulation much quicker and much easier!

A vibrator feels good on most parts of the body—head, neck, shoulders, face, hands, lower back, bottom, thighs, belly, and feet. It's very exciting when used for massaging, stimulating, and vibrating your genitals.

A vibrator vibrates with a rapid, consistent rhythm but at different speeds and intensities. Vibrators come in all shapes, sizes, colors, and styles, ranging from small cigarette-shaped models, to those resembling an erect penis. Generally they are made of plastic, rubber, or silicone.

Electric massagers, on the other hand, are generally designed to be used all over the body. They have a much stronger vibrating capacity and normally two speeds, which can also make them more noisy. Because of the intensity of the vibration, some women prefer to place fabric between themselves and the massager to cushion the vibrations, or to hold the massager to one side of the genitals, which allows the outer labia to cover and protect the clitoris. The manufacturers of electric massagers usually make no reference to their use for sexual pleasure.

The gentle or intense vibration these devices produce encourages the flow of blood to the area of the body to which they are applied. This relaxes the muscles and at the same time stimulates the sensitive nerve endings. Vibrators are most commonly used on the woman's vaginal lips—outer and inner—and particularly on the clitoris. They can also be partially inserted into the yoni, and can be used to stimulate other erogenous zones on both men and women.

The *Kama Sutra* suggests that only natural objects be used as dildos, and lists bananas, mangos, carrots, radishes, cucumbers, the stalks of plants or mushrooms, gourds and other fruits and vegetables that resemble the erect lingam in shape and texture. Nowadays, dildos are made from silicon, rubber, vinyl, or lucite for both vaginal and anal insertion. Some are amazingly lifelike with molded glans, bulging veins, and even a scrotum. They come in many colors, sizes, and shapes—straight, bent, curved, rippled, ribbed, smooth, and double-tipped or double-ended. Some have belts so you can wear them. Some dildos and vibrators are curved to reach the G-spot and to simultaneously stimulate the clitoris. You also can get lifelike renditions of flaccid penises—pliable and stretchy.

When you're using sex toys, always remember this rule for safe sex—don't put a dildo, vibrator or other toy (or a penis) into the vagina after it has been used in the anus without washing it first or covering it with a fresh condom.

WHY USE A VIBRATOR?

Why not! You won't know whether you enjoy it or not until you've tried one, and it can add a new dimension to your sex life, alone or with a lover. You can use one anywhere on your body, from your face to the soles of your feet, and its great advantage is that it can be used privately to explore what feels good for you. Discover the most pleasurable areas of your body, the best speed, intensity of pressure, duration of contact, etc. etc. etc.! Don't view sex aids as a threat to sexual intimacy but as an extra helping hand.

Vibrators can be useful when a lover is not available, or as an aid to a healthy release of sexual tension or muscular tension as required. They also can be valuable tools for spicing up or adding

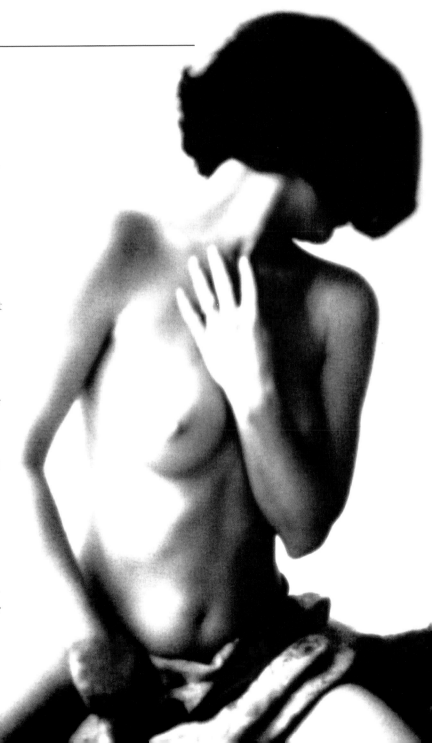

some fun to a sexual relationship that has become rather tired and predictable. Vibrators are designed primarily to stimulate the clitoris to produce an orgasm. They are equally effective and pleasurable to use during self-pleasuring and intimate sexual activity with a lover. And vibrators can be just as pleasurable for men, too.

The choice of available sex toys, massagers, and other aids has become huge, which does not make choosing any easier. I prefer the strong and more silent types such as the Hitachi Magic Wand and the Eroscillator. The Magic Wand is a massage vibrator that has become so successful that, although not originally intended for use on the genitals, attachments to stimulate the G-spot have been made for it. The Eroscillator is for external and clitoral stimulation. Both are electrically powered. Unfortunately, you cannot try before you buy, so it's pot luck or buying by recommendation. It really depends what you want from your dildo or vibrator—pleasure foremost, although where and how and what speed and texture will help to determine your choice.

According to Tantra, the direct contact between bodies has a special potency that can never be matched by substitutes. However dildos and vibrators have given people the freedom to be in control of their own sexuality. Moreover, they can help preorgasmic women, as well as improving genital muscle control to create better orgasms for some.

Many men feel they are responsible for creating the proper sexual climate with their lovers, so a man may see a woman's suggestion of using a vibrator as a sign of failure on his part. He may feel that he is being replaced by a machine or device.

To overcome these feelings, try to involve your lover in your choice and use of sex toys from the beginning. Try using your chosen sex toy on his inner thighs, between his anus and scrotum, and on the shaft of his lingam. Probably the most useful way to proceed from there is to see if he can get comfortable with the vibrator by using it on himself or by having it used on him. Then move on to both of you using it, and including it in your lovemaking.

COCK RINGS

Another device that is often effective is the penile ring or cock ring—usually a soft, fairly tight rubber, plastic, leather, or metal ring that encircles the base of the lingam. Some also encircle the testicles. A cock ring is used to encourage and maintain an erection, and works by assisting the muscles that control the flow of blood to the lingam itself, by restricting the flow of blood out of the lingam but not into it. Vibrating cock rings have a small vibrator attached, which can be positioned directly against the scrotum or lingam for a pleasant buzz and also provides pleasurable vibrations to a lover during intercourse.

Cock rings sometimes incorporate a soft extension in the form of a pad with protuberances that brush against the clitoris during intercourse. This added stimulation can help a woman to achieve orgasm. Clitoral stimulation is usually the most important part of sexual excitement for a woman, so cock rings can be useful even when the man has no problems with erection.

OTHER AIDS

Furniture can be used as a sexual aid by helping maintain new positions. Playful devices like swings and rocking chairs can add new dimensions to sex. Oils, food, and water jets from showers—in fact, any invention conceived of in the ecstasies of loving can be sex aids. Your whole environment can be thought of as a sexual aid, so take care to make it beautiful and inspiring. The human body itself has a wealth of possibilities in the limbs, hands, fingers, toes, chin, nose, breasts, and tongue.

Another essential sex aid is lubrication. Using your own or your lover's saliva is the best lubrication. However, I would also recommend any cold-pressed or unprocessed oil—pure and unadulterated—from nuts, seeds, or fruits, such as coconut, sunflower, and olive. Avoid anything that is mineral- or petroleum-based, such as baby oil, Vaseline, or petroleum jelly.

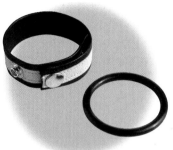

It is important to note that an oil-based lubricant will make condoms disintegrate. So, when using condoms, always use a water-based lubricant such as K-Y Jelly or Astroglide (widely available in drugstores and pharmacies).

Exotic lingerie can be fun and a great help with arousal. Open-crotch panties, peephole bras, and garter belts are exciting to wear and view. Underwear that titillates by just hiding the erotic regions can be even more sexy. Sheer, satiny fabrics, unusual colors, see-through lace, and feather trimmings all can help to add fun to foreplay. Leather, rubber, and vinyl clothes are also popular erotic apparel.

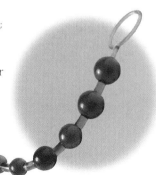

Of course, it is not necessary to spend any money at all to find sex aids; strategically placed mirrors can have a dramatic effect, a ribbon can be tied at the base of the lingam as a cock ring, or you can wear rubber or latex gloves to touch your lover. All you need is a little imagination and a willingness to get away from a routine approach to sexual activity.

SEX TOYS AND RELATIONSHIPS

As long as we think of sex as a performance, many lovers may continue to feel threatened or inadequate when their partners want to introduce a vibrator or other aid into lovemaking. If the goal is pleasure rather than performance, then the threat is removed, and sex becomes a journey of mutual discovery and intimacy.

I love my vibrator. Apart from the extraordinary pleasure I get from it, it

"Sex is man's most vibrant energy, but it should not be an end unto itself: sex should lead man to his soul. The goal is from lust to light."

OSHO

helps me to relax, boosts my creative energy, and has taught me to be more confident sexually and less dependent. It also encourages blood flow and muscle contractions in the yoni, which helps to keep it fit and healthy. However, it cannot replace the sensations of touch and love with another being.

With a sense of adventure, using a vibrator or other sex aid can free you from dependence on your lover. It can also enhance, enrich, or revitalize an already satisfying sexual relationship, or refresh and provide sexual variety in a long-term monogamous partnership or a temporarily tired relationship. It is easy, when the first flush of excitement in a new relationship is over, to fall into a jaded, repetitive sexual routine. From a lively expression of love and mutual enjoyment of one another, sex can degenerate into something close to a mildly pleasant chore.

Using some form of sex aid in these circumstances can have helpful effects far beyond the fun gained from the toy itself. Occasionally, introducing a new sex toy can help keep a sexual relationship on a stimulating and enjoyable level.

Sex is always a very personal thing, and with most aids, the attitude of the person using them is as important as the physical working of the device itself. Whether the problem is premature ejaculation or difficulty in getting and keeping an erection, or is connected with difficulty in achieving orgasms, confidence can play a crucial role. If you gain this from using an aid, then it works. What you are really finding is confidence in yourself—the sex aid is just a way to achieve it. Naturally, the best sex aid is love!

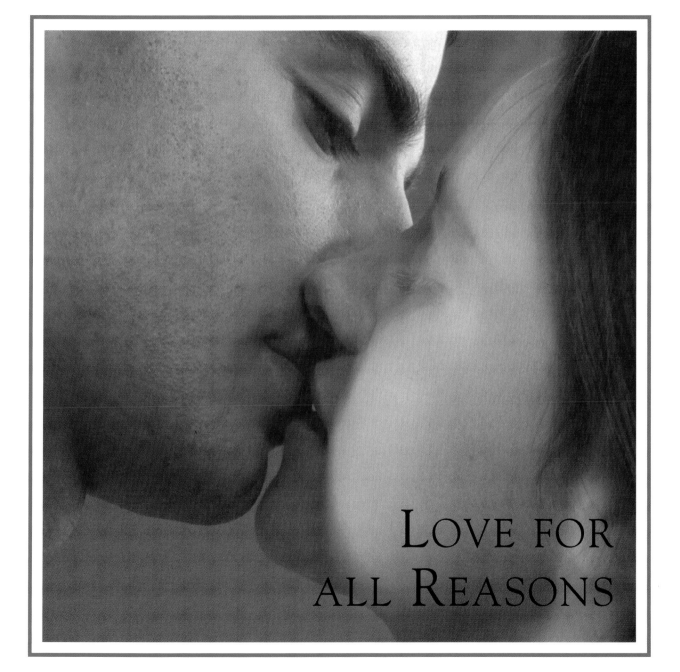

LOVE FOR
ALL REASONS

MAKING LOVE THAT LASTS

 "The only transformer and alchemist that turns everything into gold is love. The only magic against death, ageing, ordinary life, is love."

ANAÏS NIN

What if the fairy tales were concluded like this: "...and they lived happily ever after, although they had to work at it!" Marriage and intimate relationships are a journey, a process, and never easy! A marriage or sustained relationship must provide emotional satisfaction, physical satisfaction, open communication, or intellectual stimulation to keep it alive and flourishing.

I am not married and have never been married, so "How do you make love that lasts and keep making love to the same person," is a question I have posed to many married friends and to myself about my long-term relationships. There seems to be a resounding repetition of components. The most basic of these are communication, shared interests, individual interests, sexual compatibility, affection, a constructive approach to problems, forgiveness, and saying "sorry," full acceptance and appreciation of each other, mutual growth, trust, respect, zest for life and love, and occasional space from one another!

Just as lovemaking is experienced as a dance, so marriage needs to be a dialogue. Not just being able to talk to one another on a variety of subjects and to have an interest in each other's views, but also being comfortable with each other in silence.

It is not enough for a couple to love each other; they have to like each other as well. Friendships are often more enduring than marriages, so unless there is a strong element of friendship within the relationship, its foundations may be very insecure.

Having shared interests and doing some things together is important (so is having some independent interests). Often, it is common interests that bring two people together, and sometimes common interests develop within the relationship, or one partner takes up some of the interests of the other.

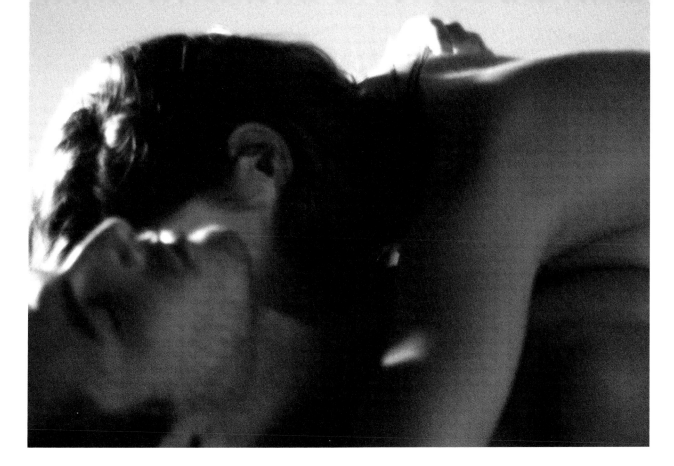

Sexual compatibility is usually a must in an enduring relationship, and remaining open to new ideas is a positive step toward keeping eroticism alive.

Appreciating and understanding that life and relationships are adventures to be enjoyed and not just "lived through" are invaluable qualities in both lovers. It is important to keep this sense alive despite problems that may arise. Hard times or bad times do not, generally, last long, and a couple who are able to keep intimate communication open, maintain a zest for life, and who seek new ways to enjoy themselves together, will be more likely to come through the hard times with their relationship intact and their intimate bonds even stronger.

In any relationship there are going to be difficulties and tensions. Conflicts and differences of opinion are bound to occur, and they must be dealt with intelligently, positively, and constructively. If they are not brought out into the open, resentment will build and trouble and disaster may follow.

Relationship Essentials

The ability to forgive yourself and your lover is an essential ingredient in any relationship. Pride is the antithesis of love. If we are too proud to say "I'm sorry," and to mean it, we are incapable of loving. Develop and nourish love through practicing care and concern for your lover.

Probably, the single most important factor of a long and successful relationship or marriage is completely accepting one another as you are, despite the inevitable faults, weaknesses, and shortcomings. The only person you can change is yourself, so you must accept your lover as he or she is and love all of that person. We all want to be loved and accepted just as we are.

Every relationship as it develops and evolves undergoes continuous examination and assessment, whether a couple are married or not. On one level, relationships can be improved by earning more money, creating a stable home, and ensuring the happiness of one's children. They can also be improved if couples are lovingly supportive of one another, reaffirm commitment to one another and the relationship, or make more time for sexual and nonsexual togetherness. On a deeper level, what most enhances a relationship is being open to a change of attitudes and supporting one

another's growth and development as individuals and as a couple, so bringing out the best in one another. This does not mean changing your lover and his or her attitudes, rather it is about being open to the possibility of changing yourself as you grow and develop. It is important to feel good with and about yourself. If you can function beautifully separately, when you come together you can create something different, something special.

Bringing out the best in each other means total acceptance of oneself and one's lover and bringing out the best qualities of the male and female energy in oneself. When two people become one in lovemaking, both momentarily lose their identities and their egos; mind is gone and time is gone.

Changes Over Time

We all need reminding about certain essential qualities to refresh and to keep our love alive in long-term relationships. Let's begin with emphasizing and acknowledging the positive in all areas of the relationship.

Whenever you are pleased with something, be sure to say so. When you appreciate something your lover has done for you, tell him or her. When you think he or she looks good, say so. Constantly reiterate your commitment to the relationship and remind yourself that everything you say and do must build toward improving, not weakening the relationship.

Our sexual activity changes as we change our views on life and as we move through its different phases. In order to bring into focus a change in attitude toward sex, couples need to communicate openly, otherwise sex remains simply as predictable sexual mechanics on a biological level and so much is missed.

To help be aware of how your relationship is developing, clarify your expectations of each other by writing down a list of expectations then exchanging and reading them occasionally. Men and women will make different decisions at different phases of their development; discuss and give consideration to those changes in yourself and your lover.

Ponder the events of your life together, and reflect on whether promises have been fulfilled, or expectations lived up to. This will help to keep the relationship alive and vital.

Give yourselves permission to ask, question, or comment on things that may help you to understand each other and yourselves better—"I've always wanted to ask you if...," "I've never told you before, I'd like you to...," "Do you know what turns me on the most...," "Which do you like better...?"

Describe the qualities that for you make a good sexual experience. Recall the sexual experiences that you have had with your lover that stand out in your mind, and see which qualities those experiences have in common. Each person's idea of what is important in a good sexual experience reflects his or her own uniqueness. Every person's approach to the world is different and each of us has our own individual idea as to which factors are necessary for a satisfying life.

Give each other the space to be honest about what you like and don't like, want and don't want. Take the initiative and do not expect your lover to intuitively know what you do and don't like—tastes change. Intimacy, communication, and patience are what you can offer to one another.

 "The fruit of all good marriages is lasting love"

KAMA SUTRA

HONESTY

If one of you feels your lovemaking is not good enough, the other will also surely feel it, too. Do not be afraid to admit to one another that your lovemaking is not good enough. Do it

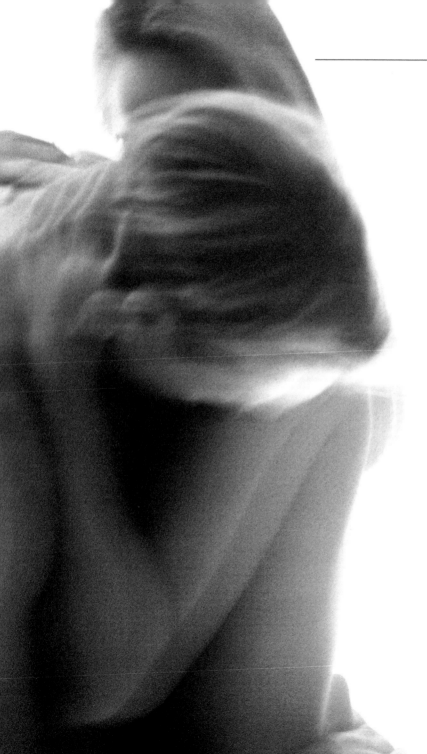

without blaming or accusing yourself or your lover. Use it as a positive way of recreating something new and different and improved together.

Love dies between lovers when you hide the truth that your lovemaking is not good enough. Resentment, dissatisfaction, and frustration build up and will eventually explode. Admit that you don't know what to do about it and admit that you cannot do it alone. When you truly surrender in humility, help is always there within you—and then it will appear outside you. Such honesty and self-knowledge generates passion, commitment, and the power of love. If you have courage and honesty and really desire your freedom, you will be living your love.

A sexual experience might feel great, and there are also times when it will not feel so great. If you remain totally open and honest and accepting of who you are and who your lover is—remaining true to yourselves—this openness is not changed because an experience is either good or bad.

The openness is unlimited and expresses itself as unconditional love, spontaneous and alive. It becomes the nature of every single moment.

An Atmosphere for Love

Grant each other the freedom that can only be built on trust. Freedom alone is the atmosphere in which true love can flourish. I want to believe that a couple who can make love ecstatically together are likely to experience for themselves, and with each other, peace, joy, and harmony in every way and in every aspect of their lives. Hence their loving attraction for each other may increase and become a more permanent one.

Years of habit may make new sexual experiences and practices seem strange and even threatening. However, fresh and novel experiences in an established, secure context can be particularly pleasing, erotic, and enticing. Said at the appropriate moment and in a warm and loving way, "Let's spice up our love life a little" can be a very positive and effective way of introducing new sexual activities to your love life. Support each other to find excitement and reintroduce variety, innovation, and surprise.

Enlivening Relationships

It is very common, after many years together, to become complacent. To avoid this, you must learn to interact with your lover in different ways. An attitude of healthy inquisitiveness and experimentation will open up whole new realms of possibilities and sensuous experiences.

Move beyond traditional sex roles. If your partner always initiates your lovemaking, you can take on this role for a while. Experiment with being receptive and assertive by being on the top and on the bottom; take turns with oral loving and erotic massage.

Making sounds, using your voices, deepening breathing, and allowing more of your bodies to become involved will also add a new dimension to your lovemaking. Experiment with the arousing pleasure of stimulating new sexual focal points.

Make time to be together in both sexual and nonsexual ways—to be loving and erotic, seductive, and flirtatious with one another—in order to bring about a welcome and exciting return to your sexual yesterdays.

Discover new ways of loving, places to love in, and times to love, perhaps with the added excitement of the possibility of getting caught. When waking up, kiss your lover. When saying goodbye, kiss your lover. When meeting after work, kiss your lover. When watching TV, cuddle up. Hug your lover as often as you can. When talking, put your arms around one another. When walking, hold your lover's hand. Kiss your lover goodnight.

A willingness to improve and keep communication open and clear, and to be considerate of your lover's feelings, is also essential. If you want to say "no" to something, say why and what you would rather do instead. If you are requesting or suggesting something your lover does not agree to, be patient and understanding. Find out why he or she feels that way. And rather than dwelling on past grievances, talk about anticipated pleasures. If you are in any doubt about your lover's meaning, intention, or desires, ask rather than guess or assume. Your interest will, generally, be appreciated.

Relate to your lover as a person, as an individual in his or her own right, rather than just as a body or your other half. Be willing to please and be pleased, to serve and be served, to give and to receive, to trust and be trusted. Be flexible, courteous, considerate, and kind. Look to find the balance between seriousness and fun, and always remember to play!

A LASTING RELATIONSHIP

There are couples who, after some years of marriage or cohabitation, no longer make love and yet still find fulfillment in their relationships. Love for them is companionship, sharing interests, enjoying family life, caring for one another. Sometimes such couples even have an agreement whereby one or both of them have their sex needs catered to outside. However, it seems to me that the most fulfilling relationships are those in which sex and love are united, just as the most enjoyable acts of lovemaking are with a loved one.

For a relationship to grow and endure, reality must balance romantic idealism. A lasting relationship requires that both partners cease building up images of themselves and their lover and accept each other for what they truly are and who they truly are. This is one of the crucial differences between loving and being in love. Mutual growth and the respect and support for one another's growth, change, and development, will bring joy in a secure relationship and create even stronger bonds as you go through life together.

Quality must come into all aspects of life, with love becoming meaningful in sex and the relationship flowering into one in which both sex and love have become significant. It is an illusion to think that each person will progress at exactly the same rate as the other. Patience, understanding, and willingness to wait, to accept whatever time it takes for both to do what they must, are what makes a marriage spiritual.

Each of us is an individual with an individual consciousness, and so everyone's development will be uniquely his or her own. However, by supporting one another and by discovering the purpose, and possibly the goals, of our individual lives—spiritually, mentally, emotionally, and physically—we can be truly together.

Two people involved in a relationship of such closeness and intensity need to support each other. Reflecting deeply each day, putting into practice what they know, and thinking before speaking, will improve the quality of any couple's life.

NEVER TOO OLD

Apparently, people in couples live longer than single people. The Taoists, who were passionately committed to the search for health and longevity, believed that in order to remain healthy and to live longer, people should make love until the day they die.

True love and sexual power, for the Taoists, is the ability to satisfy oneself and one's lover, and to do so over a lifetime. This ability increases with our understanding and acceptance of ourselves, of one another, as well as adjusting to the inevitable physiological changes that take place.

Sex, like our bodies, changes as we grow older. There are changes in our sexual responses and our sexual desires. This does not mean that sex has to diminish; on the contrary, each sexual stage and each decade of our lives offers its own unique passionate possibilities and the opportunity for a more profound relationship.

EVOLVING RELATIONSHIPS

Although a woman's fertility peaks in early adulthood, her ability for sexual pleasure can expand throughout the course of her life. For many women, menopause brings with it an increase in sexual drive. As men get older, their testosterone levels decrease whereas women's testosterone levels increase (relative to their other hormones). So, over time, men become more yin and women become more yang. The sexes actually become more compatible as they age and as their hormonal differences become less extreme.

For some men and women, after a certain age sexuality becomes an insignificant or indifferent part of life. However, most older people continue to experience some form of sexual intimacy. As we age we do not suddenly become asexual beings; our capacity for sexual intimacy will remain with us our entire lives. What does change is the way sexuality is expressed.

After years of sexual experience, expressions of sexuality and love become more refined and more evolved, and there is a depth of intimacy available as men and women deepen and cultivate their sexual energy.

As we all approach later life, certain factors are no longer necessarily as prevalent as they were, such as caring for children or following a career. This means that our personal relationships take on an increased importance. Making love is a way to affirm the love of life. It is an expression of the satisfaction gained from the present. It expresses the closeness of our deepest relationships and is an important measure of the quality of our lives.

PHYSIOLOGICAL CHANGES

Masters and Johnson showed there were certain advantages to the later years of sexual activity, provided that people understood and allowed for the changes that inevitably occurred in their sexual response cycles.

The first phase of sexual response, the excitement or arousal phase, generally takes longer in middle age than in youth. An older man will find his erection comes more slowly, the angle of his erection will have changed, and his lingam will not be as hard as it was when he was younger. However, his potential for erection is unchanged. Given time and appropriate stimulation, he may become as erect as ever.

In the plateau phase, the main advantage to being older is that the man is generally able to achieve much better control of his ejaculation. His urge to ejaculate is less intense, so he can remain in a state of pleasurable erection and stimulation for a long time. This increases his potential for experiencing

multiple orgasms without ejaculation. However, when an older man does ejaculate, the sensation may only last half as long as before and with much fewer spasms. He then loses his erection much sooner and takes much longer to have another erection.

For older women, stages of sexual response change their characteristics, too. A young woman usually produces lubrication within 15 to 30 seconds of arousal, whereas a postmenopausal woman may require several minutes. In the plateau phase, the older woman does not manifest the changes in skin color that a younger woman does, nor does her yoni canal increase in size. The experience of orgasm as vaginal contractions tends to be shorter—four to five as opposed to eight to twelve.

With the awareness and a proper understanding of the differences in sexual functioning and sexual response between young and older lovers, many worries can be dispelled. Sexual capacity does change with age, yet it need never end, and the quality of satisfaction in a loving and mature relationship can more than compensate for the quantity and frequency enjoyed in youth.

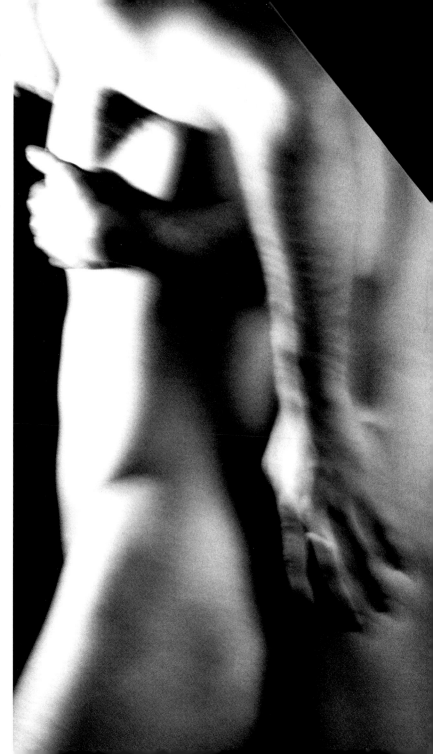

KEEPING IN SEXUAL SHAPE

Our sex organs, like all our other organs, need regular exercise in order to stay strong and healthy. Continuance of loving sexual activity helps keep the entire physical organism vigorous and in tone, and greatly contributes to general good health and a sense of well-being.

Nobody likes to feel too old for love. Those who can continue to feel, whatever their age, that they can love and be loved are a long way toward escaping the terrible sense of loneliness and isolation many older people suffer. In some individuals the urge to make love diminishes, but there is no reason why men and women cannot continue to make love right through their lives. It may just need some adapting.

MENOPAUSE AND VIROPAUSE

"The most creative force in the world is the menopausal woman with zest."

MARGARET MEAD

Menopause is the cessation of reproductive functioning in a woman—not the cessation of sexual functioning. The two systems that include the sexual organs—the reproductive and the sexual system— contribute to the mental and emotional health and psychological development of the individual, and are entirely independent of one another.

Menopause brings with it diminishing estrogen, which for some women is the start of an emotional roller coaster. Common symptoms include irritability, depression, mood swings, headaches, hot flashes, night sweats, palpitations, disturbed sleep, inability to concentrate, along with many physical and emotional changes.

For some women, sexual penetration becomes less desirable because there is less elasticity, the opening of the yoni can become smaller, the vaginal tissue can become thinner and more delicate, and less natural lubrication is produced. However, if you are in good physical and emotional health, staying sexual, whether by self-pleasuring or by intercourse with a lover, will help to alleviate many of these symptoms. Like every other part of the body, your sexual organs need exercise to remain healthy; menopause need not be a reason to give up on your sexuality.

Exercising the PC muscle (see page 54) and keeping it toned will also help. The exercise will promote blood flow to your pelvic region and energy flow to the sexual organs, and it will also help keep your bladder control strong and effective.

Betty Dodson, in *Sex for One*, writes, "I am convinced it's important to continue doing some kind of penetration to slough off dead cells, aerate the vaginal barrel, stimulate natural lubrication, moisturize the vagina with natural oils, increase hormone levels with regular orgasms, and keep the PC muscle toned. This not only keeps us sexual, it also prevents the seepage of urine."

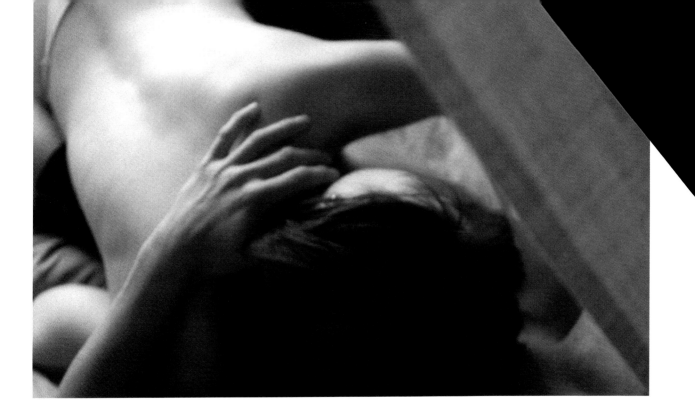

VIROPAUSE

Men undergo a similar sexual experience to menopause called viropause. This is the time during an older man's life when his levels of the hormones testosterone and DHEA (dehydroepiandrosterone) start to decrease more rapidly.

A man doesn't necessarily know when he is going through viropause. It can happen without him realizing, and it may coincide with a time in his life—the so-called "midlife crisis"—when he begins to reflect on his past and question his future.

POSITIVE AGEING

The relationship between lovers is the beginning of a journey, not the end, and long-term relationships can be vibrant, alive, emotional, fun, and sexy. According to Taoists, it takes years to reach the heights of physical, emotional, and spiritual union. Seven years to know your lover's body, seven years to know your lover's mind, and seven years to know your lover's spirit. The longer we share ourselves with our lovers, the better we know each other and the stronger and more intimate our bonds can be. Love is not based on your lovemaking techniques and how many orgasms you have, but on the quality of love and loving you experience together.

We need to embrace our entire sexual life-cycle with positive images of growing older. Menopause and viropause can be times of power with renewed self-confidence, energy, inner beauty, and sexual abundance. Some men and women will rely on masturbation for their orgasms. Some will enjoy the comfort of familiar sex with a loving partner, and some, men and women, will have their first erotic affair with another woman or another man. A few will be relieved to let go of all forms of sex altogether, and some will take younger lovers.

By honoring and celebrating this phase of our lives, we can change our own and society's perceptions of growing older, and embrace and respect ourselves as Elders, Healers, Holders of Wisdom, Guides, and Teachers.

SUGGESTIONS FOR LOVE THAT LASTS

- Be sexual with one another or with yourself by self-pleasuring at least once a week. This will boost the blood flow to your sexual organs to keep them healthy and strong, and it will also keep your hormones primed.
- Touch each other often. Loving affection produces the hormone oxytocin and we instantly feel better for it.
- For older men and women making love—give the man plenty of genital stimulation and use the soft entry technique when needed (see page 44). Reduce the number of times he ejaculates.
- Make sure the woman is well-lubricated.
- Avoid or reduce cigarettes, alcohol, and any drugs that have negative sexual side effects.

- Exercise daily to keep active and flexible.
- Eat fresh and healthy foods.
- Free yourself of expectations during lovemaking and you will avoid dissatisfaction and frustration. Explore with joy in a spirit of adventure and playfulness.
- Accept that not every love encounter you share will be a masterpiece. Keep your excitement high and your expectations low.
- Avoid taking yourselves or the practices too seriously. Play with each other and you will experience your lovemaking as fun as well as profound.

LUST OR LOVE?

Sexual attraction is a lifelong powerful current that either adds energy and magnetism to relationships or remains a constantly disrupting influence, depending on our skill and awareness of directing it.

The more complete and balanced the combination of love, liking, and lust, the greater the degree of emotional and physical letting-go into truly transforming loving. If lust is transcended, sex can become love. When sex is just a mechanical urge you will never feel truly fulfilled, not because of the sex, but because of the "mechanicalness" of the sex. The best sex comes from allowing rather than doing—allowing the sexual energy between you to move as it desires.

Fast food is quick, easy, and looks better than it tastes. The same is also true for some fast sex, particularly if that is all you have and experience. However, if you can sustain the quality of love and care toward your lover, as well as enjoy having quick, spontaneous, lusty sex, then there is no problem. But just as maintaining a diet of fast food will ultimately be disappointing, the same can be true of fast sex.

Inevitably there will be times when you will not have the appetite for prolonged lovemaking. Don't let that be because you have never tried it! Undoubtedly once a couple have fully experienced making love, they will rarely be bored or tired of it. It is experienced as a complete pleasure, not as a strain or effort, or a chore. In fact, it can prove to be an energizing experience for both the man and woman, particularly if the man can withhold his ejaculation.

 "Change base lust into refined love and it is worth more than a mountain of gold."

IKKYU

Prolonged lovemaking does not necessarily mean spending the whole day in bed—though if you can, then why not! Of course, the intensity of lovemaking will vary from time to time. Most couples probably spend more time watching television or sitting in front of a computer than physically sharing love with one another.

DON'T HURRY SEX!
Choose your moments and kindle the flame when making love. If you are hurried in everything you will probably

be hurried in sex and love, too, as if time is being wasted. Sex is not something you can hurry, unless it is completely without love. If you hurry it you miss the very point of it. Savor and enjoy it because through it you can experience timelessness. All great things need slowness and patience so that you can become saturated. Let love be something special. Do not hurry to get to the end; forget the end completely and stay with the beginning. Remain in the present going nowhere, and melt.

Lust is a vital part of your life-force energy. To be fully appreciated, it needs to be connected to your love for your lover and cultivated, transformed, and expressed as love and compassion for yourself and for your lover. To fulfill the body's sexual needs, love turns into lust and love is interpreted as physical desire. In this way its divinity is tarnished, and emotional needs for love become secondary to the instinctual need for sex.

So in the practice of love we have to be willing to open our hearts to emotional connection with our lover rather than staying stuck in the satisfaction of our physical and emotional needs. Wallowing in unthinking sexual desire, in pleasure without love, can be just as limiting as wallowing in pain if we do not allow ourselves to open our hearts.

Whether you choose to give in to your lustful urges and make love quickly, or choose to make love a prolonged experience, only approach sex when you are cheerful and full of love, when your heart is full of joy and peace and gratitude. Then your lovemaking can be prayerful, mindful, and sacred.

Nothing is wrong with pure simple sex. Imbue it with love, opening your heart, and through pure simple sex you will experience something extraordinary. It becomes a deep and intimate communication with your lover and can be experienced as playful as well as prayerful. When you are just having sex only your genitals will meet. When you are making love, a circle is created where you become one and you will feel more energetic, more alive, and more charged with the flow of energy you have created.

PASSIONATE LOVING

Lusty sex, free from constraint and pressure, is normal and fine. Sexual desire is a reflection of your energy. Loving is at its best when it is at its most flexible. Any kind of sex is acceptable provided that it is self-liberating, other-enriching, honest, faithful, responsible, life-serving, and joyous. There are times when all you want is to abandon yourself to the fun of wild and spontaneous sex. And there

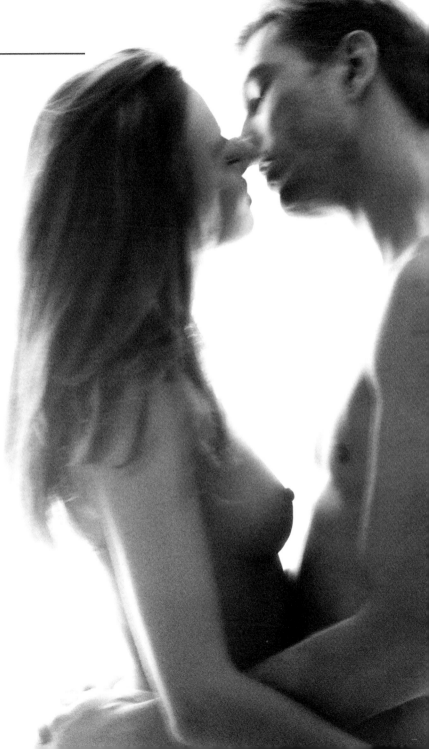

can be nothing more erotic than being
so possessed in the moment with desire
for one another that you have to do it,
have it there and then. There is also
something very exciting about the
spontaneity of it and the wildness of
your desire and fury of excitement.

However you choose to express your
passion, give love through it. Use your
whole mind, body, and spirit as a vehicle
for revealing your love. Ravish and be
vulnerable, give love through the
wildness of your desire, turn your
fury of excitement into heart-focused
love. Move in your desire with full
consciousness, because in doing that
you transcend it.

Remember love and breathe love and
open your hearts through the lust of
your desire. When you caress your lover
become the caress, when you kiss your
lover become the kiss, when you
embrace your lover, become the
embrace. Relax into non-separation.
Dissolve into the act; become love!

Let your hearts melt and relax in
deep love as your bodies rage in the
wildness of passionate sex. Transform
your lust into an expression of love. You
can enjoy yourself sexually without love
and be physically satisfied, but only with
love can you be truly fulfilled.

LOVE IN NATURE

"We belong to the ground. It is our power and we must stay close to it or maybe we will get lost."

YIRALLA

Nature perpetuates its species through sex and human beings perpetuate their species through sex. There is no getting away from it. We are surrounded by it. Everything about Nature is sexy. And everything in Nature is connected and works together in harmony. All the elements, earth, air, fire, and water; the sky and its planets, moons, and stars; the trees, plants, animals, insects, birds, and fish. We exist as part of Nature, part of the universe and cosmos, and cannot be separate from it and so are affected by all of it. Everything in the universe is contained within our own bodies. We are a microcosm, a miniature representation of the universe, the macrocosm.

The ancient Taoists believed that sexual harmony puts one in communion with the infinite force of Nature, which they saw as having sexual overtones. Earth, for instance, was the female, or yin element, and Heaven the male, or yang. The interaction between these two constitutes the whole, just as

the union of man and woman creates a oneness. And one is as important as the other. Male and female cannot be considered separately; they form a complementary, alternating whole. One defines the existence of the other.

Older indigenous cultures, who lived closer to the earth and practiced rituals tied to the cycles of Nature, were more in tune with the natural rhythms and feminine essence of the earth and life than our modern "civilized" society. Their less-complicated existence and natural belief in the divine nature of plants, animals, elements, and life itself allowed them to be more intimately acquainted with the sensuality and sexuality that dwelt within them and the forces of Nature around them. They saw sex and sexuality as a natural part of creation and as the sacred energy of life.

Pre-patriarchal religions honored fertility, creation, and sexuality in their ceremonies and rituals as different aspects of the same divine force. The pagan rites of Beltane, for example, were an offering to the earth's fertility in spring, and the solstice rites celebrated the planting and reaping of crops as a gift from the sensual, abundant body of the earth as goddess. These early people innately understood that the power and divine sexuality of the feminine principle was inherent not only in the earth, the elements, and the animals but also in their own sex organs and instincts, in the smells and tastes of their bodies, and in the natural pattern of their lives.

Gradually over time the spiritual bond between humans and the earth has been broken, the earth exploited, plundered, and desecrated. The way most of us live is cut off from our natural environment, and the materials we use in our buildings and roads block the flow of the earth's energies to our beings. We have become isolated from the earthly and celestial energies that connect us to Nature and to the world around us.

There is a great need for us as human beings to identify our sexuality with the primary forces of the universe. We need to harmonize our sexual polarity, energy, and behavior so that our human sexuality can reflect a new and positive power, beauty, and understanding, which in turn can beneficially affect Nature and the living world around us.

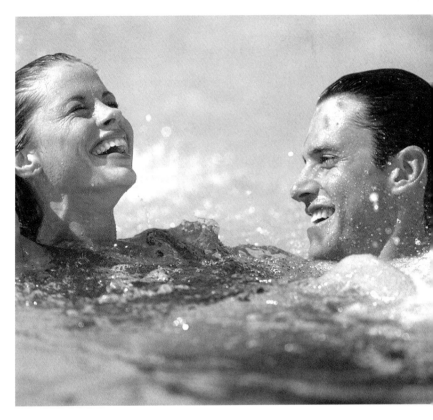

SEX AS RELIGION

In ancient cultures with matriarchal religions, sex was considered something ennobling and uplifting. Sex could take you closer to the gods rather than alienate you from them. There were many sexual rites celebrated throughout the year, in tune with the seasons of time and the rhythms of Nature. Many of these celebrations are still with us today, but they have now lost their sexual connotations.

One of these converted pagan holidays is St. Valentine's Day, taken from the ancient Roman fertility festival of Lupercalia. The Lupercalia celebrations were noted for their wild, sensual dances and lascivious orgies. Another sexual celebration was May Day. This holiday used to be celebrated by great sexual frolics around that giant phallic symbol, the maypole. The maypole represented the god's phallus in Mother Earth. People decorated it and danced around it. Raising the maypole was a symbolic sexual act. The pole represented the lingam of the god, and the hole it entered was the yoni of the Earth Goddess. By raising the maypole, the villagers symbolically fertilized Mother Earth's body so that she would be fruitful during the growing season and provide a bountiful harvest.

After the erection, decoration, and dances around the maypole, the villagers continued their May celebrations and they would have had sex with anyone willing in the ploughed fields in order to insure the fertility of the land and a prosperous yield of crops. May was a month of sexual freedom throughout rural Europe up to the 16th century. Marriage bonds were suspended for the month of May and began again in June—hence the popularity of June weddings.

NATURE'S EROTICISM

Lovemaking in a natural environment is a totally different experience to making love indoors. Natural environments can be very erotically stimulating as there is natural Shakti energy (female creative force) inherent in all the creations of Nature. With awareness and sensitivity, a couple can connect with this natural force and use their physical love to commune with the forces and elements of Nature and experience a kind of mystical communion.

Also, the unconventional and spontaneous aspects of love can be reawakened by making love in the country or on the beach. Nature and natural surroundings please the senses and put us in harmony with our spirit.

It is important to maintain contact with natural elements, not least of all because the five physical senses are the instruments of lovers and the doorway to inner eroticism.
Cultivate a sensual paradise around you, an erotic garden to sustain and enrich your sexual loving life.
- Focus on being fully in your body and using all your instincts and awakening all your sensations, to feel the pulse of the earth and Nature around you.

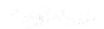

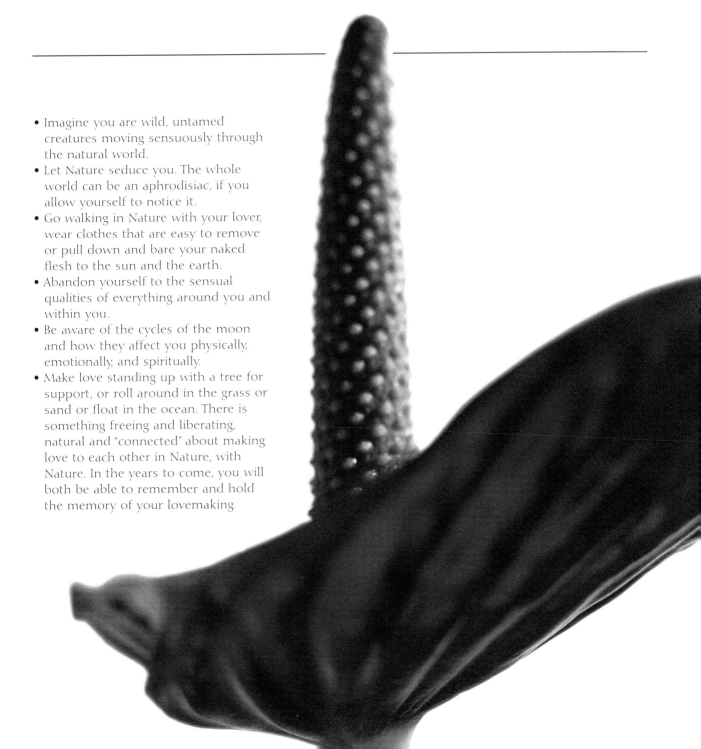

- Imagine you are wild, untamed creatures moving sensuously through the natural world.
- Let Nature seduce you. The whole world can be an aphrodisiac, if you allow yourself to notice it.
- Go walking in Nature with your lover, wear clothes that are easy to remove or pull down and bare your naked flesh to the sun and the earth.
- Abandon yourself to the sensual qualities of everything around you and within you.
- Be aware of the cycles of the moon and how they affect you physically, emotionally, and spiritually.
- Make love standing up with a tree for support, or roll around in the grass or sand or float in the ocean. There is something freeing and liberating, natural and "connected" about making love to each other in Nature, with Nature. In the years to come, you will both be able to remember and hold the memory of your lovemaking

under the stars, in the fields, or in the water as a special token of your enduring feelings for each other.

- If you are a menstruating woman, be aware if your menstruation is tied in with the cycles of the moon. Do you menstruate at the time of the full moon or the new moon?

- Reconnect yourself to the infinite force of Nature. Keep your sensual self alive and tantalized all the time.

- Admire, and play with erotic objects found in Nature. I have the most exquisite and perfect phallus formed from coral and the outline and shape of a yoni also formed from coral. They sit on my altar and remind me of the glorious wonders of Nature.

- Feathers, plants, and flowers are a sensual delight for the eyes and the skin. Aroma is another powerful stimulus for the senses—inhale deeply the earth, air, fruits, and the musky aromas of sex and flowers.

- Notice the erotic qualities of Nature. A bumblebee plunging into a gorgeous flower, the exquisite colors of a vivid sunset, the sight and sound of ocean waves, the sight of green rolling hills or craggy mountain peaks. Rub the earth in your hands, let it fall through your fingers, caress your body with the petals of a flower, eat a blade of grass. Close your eyes and let the sounds around you wash over you.

- Introduce natural elements into your home—plants and flowers, a shell picked up from the beach where you made love, or a pebble or stone from the field you lay down in.

- Fill your home with flowers. Enjoy their beauty, inhale their fragrance, garnish your food with them, float them in your bath, scatter their petals over your bed.

- See and acknowledge the living spirit in all things. Be filled with respect, awe, wonder, and love for the sacred in everything. Rocks, streams, trees, animals, clouds–every living thing. When you become conscious of every flower, shell, fruit, and seed as a living essence of sensuality and beauty, they will come alive for you and reveal their richness in their colors, smells, textures, tastes, and sounds.

- Be aware of what you see, feel, hear, and smell, and the taste in your mouth. The space, the sounds, the smells around you, and even your own breathing. Being open to all that will gradually turn you on to life, to love, to all of it, more and more.

PRO CREATION

The common view that the main purpose of sexuality and sexual desire is simply for reproduction is unique to Western philosophy and science, and barely 300 years old. This view was probably the result of puritanical religions, which sought to divorce people's sexuality from their spiritual development.

Among many tribal peoples, reproduction is considered a possible outcome of sexual activity, it is not regarded as the basis of sexual desire. Eastern philosophies held that sexual love had a higher form and purpose. They regarded human sexuality and sexual desire as vehicles to reach other levels of consciousness and experience as well as for procreation. Lovemaking, like meditation, has the potential to release us from our thought processes and allow us to feel a transcendental energy within our own bodies.

Of all the aspects of being human, sex is the most neglected, which seems absurd when you think that it is sex on which the procreation of life depends, and on which new souls entering the world depend. It is vital that we succeed in bringing harmony to the act of sex, and that we recognize it as a form of sacred communion. In this way a better humanity can come into being.

In Nature, everything pivots on reproduction to assure the continuity of life. Sex is divine. It is the primal energy of sex that creates new life and that is the most mysterious force of all. In the union of the lingam and yoni that divinity, the power to create, becomes visible in humanity. So by conscious loving and honoring, conception and birthing can take on a whole new and profound significance.

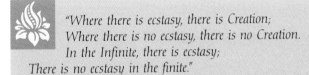

"Where there is ecstasy, there is Creation;
Where there is no ecstasy, there is no Creation.
In the Infinite, there is ecstasy;
There is no ecstasy in the finite."

CHANDOGYA UPANISHAD

MINDFUL CONCEPTION

Conceiving a child is a serious matter that requires great thought and great preparation. The parents need to eat well, be of good health, think positively, and be surrounded by peaceful environments.

Creating your own ritual for conscious lovemaking with the possibility of conception can be a wonderful and very powerful way of

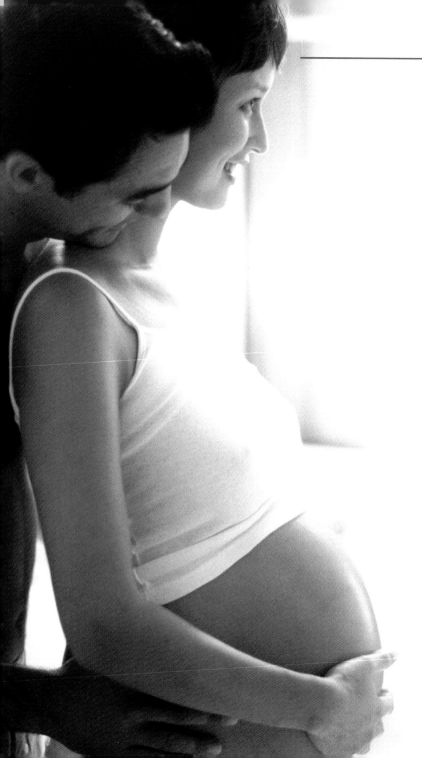

bringing new life into the world. Consider yourselves as indulging in an act of ultimate love as well as in an act of procreation.

RITUAL FOR CONCEPTION

When you feel the time has arrived for conceiving a child, take a relaxing bath together. Then create a pleasant, restful, and inspiring space with a comfortable room temperature, a candle or two burning, a little incense or perfume, and some soothing background music.

Allow at least 30 minutes after your bath before you begin to make love. Use the time to honor, nurture, and cherish one another with kisses and caresses. Be totally present together in conscious physical union. Maintain eye contact and be aware of your breathing. Gazing into one another's eyes is a powerful way of connecting while making love and can be challenging as well as inviting. Accept your sexuality and lovemaking as a form of sacred communion. After you have made love, stay joined together. This is a precious time and will strengthen the bonds of your intimacy.

In *The Tao of Sexology*, Stephen T. Chang quotes the Taoists, who say that if a couple plan to have a child, it is absolutely essential that they take great care, at the time of the conception and throughout pregnancy, to ensure that the child will be totally healthy. The

Taoists believe it is the responsibility of the parents to ensure that succeeding generations are strong and healthy.

To ensure a child's health, they recommend that the following rules be adhered to:

- Do not conceive a child if either parent is drunk or alcoholic at the time of the conception.
- Do not conceive a child when either parent is extremely tired.
- Do not conceive a child in wartime or while there is any struggle going on, whether at the place of a parent's work or at home within the family.
- Do not conceive during severe weather conditions, for instance during a hurricane or violent storm.
- Do not conceive during a sunset.
- Do not conceive when either parent is under the influence of drugs or medication. This includes smoking.

CHOOSING THE SEX OF A CHILD

The theory behind sex selection is that in a woman's cervix and uterus there are highly acidic fluids, which are neutralized during orgasm by alkaline secretions. The sperms carrying the male chromosome are slower than those carrying the female chromosome. They are also more-resilient survivors of acidic conditions in the cervix and uterus than the sperms carrying the female chromosome.

TO CONCEIVE A MALE CHILD

Lovemaking must be brief and the man must ejaculate before the woman has an orgasm. The man must withdraw his lingam halfway before ejaculating.

The thinking behind this technique is that by ejaculating very quickly with shallow penetration, the man lengthens the distance the sperms have to travel. The sperms carrying the female chromosomes, which swim faster than those carrying the male chromosomes, then contact, die in, and neutralize the strong acidic secretions before the sperms carrying the male chromosomes arrive. So the chances of a sperm carrying the male chromosome fertilizing the egg are increased.

TO CONCEIVE A FEMALE CHILD

To conceive a female child, the man must bring the woman through many orgasms before he ejaculates while penetrating deeply. Deep penetration reduces the distance the sperm has to travel, so the chances for conceiving a girl are increased. And because orgasms produce acid-neutralizing alkaline secretions, they increase the chance of a sperm with the female chromosome fertilizing the egg.

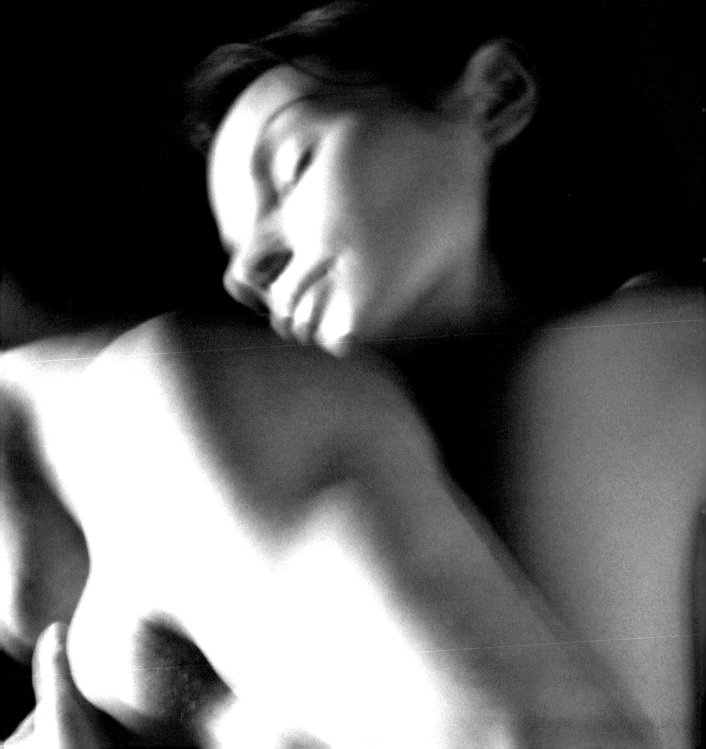

INDEX

H I J K

L M N

FURTHER READING

ABRAMS, DOUGLAS & ABRAMS, RACHEL, MD
*The Multi-Orgasmic Couple by Mantak Chia &
Maneewan Chia*
HarperSanFrancisco, 2000

BIDDULPH, STEVE AND SHAARON
*How Love Works: How to Stay in Love as a
Couple and Be True to Yourself...Even With Kids*
Thorsons, London, 2000

CAMPHAUSEN, RUFUS C. (quoted on p 46)
*The Yoni: Sacred Symbol of Female
Creative Power*
Inner Traditions, Rochester, Vermont, 1996

CHALKER, REBECCA
The Clitoral Truth
Seven Stories Press, New York, 2000

CHANG, JOLAN (quoted on p 42)
The Tao of Love & Sex
Wildwood House, Hampshire, England, 1977

CHANG, DR. STEPHEN T. (quoted on pp 58, 61)
The Tao of Sexology
Tao Publishing, San Francisco, 1986

CLAIRE, OLIVIA ST
Unleashing the Sex Goddess in Every Woman
Harmony Books, New York, 1996

DANIELOU, ALAIN (translator) (quoted on p 64)
The Complete Kama Sutra
Park Street Press, Rochester, Vermont, 1994

DANIELOU, ALAIN (quoted on p 28)
*The Phallus: Sacred Symbol of Male
Creative Power*
Inner Traditions, Rochester, Vermont, 1995

DEIDA, DAVID (quoted on pp 20, 77, 78)
*Dear Lover: A Woman's Guide to Enjoying
Love's Deepest Bliss*
Plexus, Austin, Texas, 2002
Finding God Through Sex
Plexus, Austin, Texas, 2002

Intimate Communion
Health Communications Inc, Florida, 1995
Naked Buddhism
Plexus, Austin, Texas, 2002

DODSON, BETTY, PH.D. (quoted on p 116)
Sex For One: The Joy of Selfloving
Crown Trade Paperbacks, New York, 1996

DOUGLAS, NIK AND SLINGER, PENNY (quoted on
pp 16, 31, 88, 89, 93, 154)
Sexual Secrets: The Alchemy of Ecstasy
Destiny Books, Rochester, Vermont, 1979

FEMINIST WOMEN'S HEALTH CENTERS, THE
FEDERATION OF
A New View of a Woman's Body
Feminist Health Press, Los Angeles, 1991

HARVEY, ANDREW AND MATOUSEK, MARK
Dialogues with a Modern Mystic
Quest Books, Wheaton, Illinois, 1994

LAWLOR, ROBERT (quoted on pp 98, 148)
Earth Honouring: The New Male Sexuality
Inner Traditions, Rochester, Vermont, 1989

RADHA, SWAMI SIVANANDA
*From The Mating Dance to the Cosmic Dance:
Sex, Love and Marriage from a Yogic Viewpoint*
Timeless Books, Spokane, Washington, 1992

RAMSDALE, DAVID AND ELLEN
*Sexual Energy Ecstasy: A Practical Guide to
Lovemaking Secrets of the East and West*
Bantam Books, New York, 1993

RUIZ, DON MIGUEL (quoted on p 24)
The Mastery of Love
Amber Allen Publishing, San Rafael, 1999

SUDO, PHILIP TOSHIO
Zen Sex: The Way of Making Love
HarperSanFrancisco, 2000

ACKNOWLEDGMENTS

I would like to acknowledge with
immense gratitude and love everyone in
my life, they have all been, and are,
incredible teachers for me. I thank
friends, family, and lovers for the
wisdom they impart and the love and
support they give; and all of those who
were willing to share with me the
pleasure and sometimes the pain of
their intimate sexual relationships and
their personal experiences of love and
loving. I would like to thank Sarah for
coming up with the title, and most of all
I would like to thank Torquil—whom I
love—completely.

Caroline Aldred

Carroll & Brown would like to thank:
Illustrator Amanda Williams
IT support Paul Stradling, Nicky Rein
Production Karol Davies, Nigel Reed
Picture research Sandra Schneider
Photographic assistance David Yems

Picture credits
Pages 30, 42, 47, 61, 91, 97, 144
Powerstock
Page 118 Getty Images
Page 127 Patricia
McDonough/Photonica
Page 151 Flowerphotos/Victoria
Gomez